Vegan Coo Plant Based Eating And Green Smoothies

Learn How to Quickly and Easily Prepare Vegan Meals, How to Eat a Gluten-Free Diet and How to Make Green Smoothies For Energy and Health

By Paul Dillow

© **Copyright 2020 - All rights reserved.**

The content contained within this book may not be reproduced, duplicated or transmitted without direct written permission from the author or the publisher.

Under no circumstances will any blame or legal responsibility be held against the publisher or author for any damages, reparation, or monetary loss due to the information contained within this book. Either directly or indirectly.

Legal Notice:

This book is copyright protected. This book is only for personal use. You cannot amend, distribute, sell, use, quote or paraphrase any part, or the content within this book, without the consent of the author or publisher.

Disclaimer Notice:

Please note the information contained within this document is for educational and entertainment purposes only. All effort has been executed to present accurate, up to date and reliable, complete information. No warranties of any kind are declared or implied. Readers acknowledge that the author is not engaging in the rendering of legal, financial, medical or professional advice. The content within this book has been derived from various sources. Please consult a licensed professional before attempting any techniques outlined in this book.

By reading this document, the reader agrees that under no

circumstances is the author responsible for any losses, direct or indirect, which are incurred as a result of the use of information contained within this document, including, but not limited to, —errors, omissions, or inaccuracies.

Contents:

- INTRODUCTION to Vegan Cooking Essentials 1
  - WHAT IS VEGAN COOKING? 1
  - SO, WHAT IS VEGANISM? 2
  - WHAT MAKES A CERTAIN FOOD VEGAN? 2
  - WHAT THIS BOOK IS ABOUT 4
- CHAPTER 1: COMMON INGREDIENTS 6
  - REPLACING EGGS 7
  - WHAT DO EGGS DO IN THE RECIPE? 7
  - EGG REPLACEMENT OPTIONS 7
    - Pureed Bananas 8
    - Ground Flaxseeds 8
    - Egg Replacement Product 9
    - Try Tofu 10
    - Utilizing Flour and Other Leavening Agents 11
    - Discovering the Right Egg Substitute 12
  - REPLACING MILK 13
  - REPLACING BUTTERMILK IN RECIPES 15
  - REPLACING LARD AND BUTTER 16
  - COMMON INGREDIENTS 18
  - SOY PRODUCTS 19

- WHOLE GRAINS. 23
- SEEDS AND NUTS..24
- LEGUMES 25
- VEGETABLES AND FRUITS. 26
- CANNED AND PACKAGED FOODS. 27
- INGREDIENTS TO WATCH OUT FOR 28
- INGREDIENTS FROM ANIMALS. 29
- INGREDIENTS THAT MAY BE FROM ANIMALS 32

CHAPTER 2: THE VEGAN PANTRY..35
- STEP ONE 35
- STEP TWO 36
- STEP THREE 37
- EXAMPLE 38
- BREAKFAST ITEMS 39
- SNACKS 39
- MISC. ITEMS 40
- GRAIN PRODUCTS. 40
- DRESSINGS. 41
- BAKING PRODUCTS..41

CHAPTER 3: VEGAN COOKING FUNDAMENTALS...........43
- SETTING UP YOUR KITCHEN..45
- HOW TO FOLLOW RECIPES...47
- COOKING TECHNIQUES 48
- DISCOVER HOW TO UTILIZE YOUR KNIVES 48

HEATING, BOILING AND SIMMERING 49
BAKING AND BROILING 50
HOW TO UTILIZE ALL OF YOUR APPLIANCES 50
COMMON COOKING TERMS AND WHAT THEY MEAN
.... 51

CHAPTER 4: A COMPLETE MEAL 54
CONSIDERATIONS 54
GETTING AMPLE PROTEIN 55
EATING AMPLE IRON 56
FOODS ABUNDANT IN B-VITAMINS 57
GETTING AMPLE CALCIUM 57
GETTING IT RIGHT 58
VEGAN-FRIENDLY ETHNIC CUISINE 59

CHAPTER 5: SPECIAL CONSIDERATIONS 63
DIABETES 64
CIRCULATORY DISEASES 64
LOW-FAT DIET 65
LOW SUGAR COOKING 66
LOW SODIUM COOKING 66
GLUTEN-FREE COOKING 67

CHAPTER 6: RECIPES 69
APPETIZERS 69
   Bruschetta 69
   Black Olive Hummus 71

- SOUPS 72
  - Greek-Style Chickpea Soup 72
  - Classic Minestrone Soup 73
- SALADS 75
  - Vegan Cesar Salad 75
  - Traditional Salad 76
- MAIN COURSES 77
  - Vegan Lentil Tacos 77
  - Healthy Vegetable Casserole 78
- SIDE DISHES 79
- DESSERTS 81
  - Vegan Brownies 81
- THINGS TO DO WITH FRESH FRUIT 82
- CONCLUSION of Vegan Cooking Essentials 84
- Introduction to Gluten-Free Eating 87
- Chapter 1-- What is Gluten? 90
- Chapter 2—Why All the Fuss? 94
  - 1. Celiac Disease 94
  - 2. Gluten Sensitivity 96
  - 3. Gluten Intolerance 98
- Chapter 3-- How to Diagnose Gluten Sensitivity, Celiac Disease and Gluten Intolerance 99
  - Celiac Disease Diagnosis 100
  - Diagnosing Gluten Intolerance or Gluten Sensitivity 101

- Drawbacks of the Medical System 101

Chapter 4-- How to Make it Easier for Your Physician to Make a Diagnosis 103
- Keep a Food Journal 104
- Write Down Your Signs 105
- Inform your Physician of Other Medical Conditions 106
- Inform your Physician of the Medical History of Your Family 107
- Be on Time For Your Session 108
- Have Patience 109

Chapter 5-- What are the Good Things About Gluten-Free Life? 111

Chapter 6-- Risks of Gluten-Free Eating 118

Chapter 7-- How to Delight In Gluten-Free Eating 125

Chapter 8-- So … What Should You Eat 131

Chapter 9-- Simple Gluten-Free Options 136

Conclusion of Gluten-Free Eating 140

Chapter 1: Smoothies Can Change Your Life 144
- Why We Require Nutrients 145
- Issue With Contemporary Diets 148
- Why Empty Calories Are Bad 150
- Why Smoothies Are So Good 151
- What To Anticipate When You Start With Smoothies 154

Chapter 2: The Downsides and Dangers of Smoothies 157

How to Prevent Harming Yourself With the Sugar in Smoothies 161

Chapter 3: Making the Perfect Smoothie 163

The Essentials 164

Liquid 164

Base 166

The Ratios 168

Start Mixing! 169

How to Obtain More From Your Smoothies 170

Include Garnishes 170

Sweeteners 171

Chapter 4: Fitting Smoothies Into Your Regimen ... 172

What You Need 173

Preparation and Pick-Up 175

Easy Smoothies 177

Bought Smoothie 177

Chapter 5: Energy and Defence Smoothies 179

Morning Wakeup Smoothie 180

Stress Buster Smoothie 186

Brain Fuel Smoothie 189

Breakfast Smoothie 192

Chapter 6: Smoothies for Sleep, Digestion and Hangover .. 196

The Bed Time Smoothie 197

Hangover Smoothie 200

How to Make a Smoothie For Better Food Digestion 203

Chapter 7: Smoothies for Weight-loss, Bodybuilding and Functionality 207

    The Cross Country Smoothie 207

    Bodybuilding Smoothie 210

    Fat Burning Smoothie 211

Conclusion of Green Smoothie Cleanss 214

Thank you for buying this book and I hope that you will find it useful. If you will want to share your thoughts on this book, you can do so by leaving a review on the Amazon page, it helps me out a lot.

Vegan Cooking Essentials

A Step-by-Step Guide to the Basics of Vegan Cooking and Ingredients Which You Need to Prepare Simple, Quick and Healthy Vegan Recipes

By Paul Dillow

INTRODUCTION to Vegan Cooking Essentials

WHAT IS VEGAN COOKING?

Individuals in our contemporary society are worrie about several problems. Environment and health are 2 huge ones which are at the forefront. Individuals wish to eat well and reduce their environmental impact. Dangers of obesity and global warming are 2 of the greatest worries.

Certain individuals decide that they wish to deal with both simultaneously. Making a choice to end up being a vegan is a choice which is made just as much for health reasons, along with ethical and environmental ones.

Vegan cooking is merely food which is prepared inside the vegan requirements so that it supports that way of life.

SO, WHAT IS VEGANISM?

Veganism is a vegetarianism subset. There are a number of various types. Certain vegetarians still eat eggs and/or drink milk. Not vegans, however. They are the strictest type and do not consider ANY animal products in their diet plan.

It is, without a doubt, the toughest type since individuals take a great deal of things for granted. Milk and eggs, for instance, are common baking components. So, substitutions have to be made for a vegan to have the ability to enjoy baked goods.

WHAT MAKES A CERTAIN FOOD VEGAN?

In order for food to be strictly vegan, it has to abide by specific requirements. It is necessary to keep in mind that there are a great deal of concealed ingredients in foods. It is particularly crucial to keep an eye out for these if you will pursue a vegan diet plan.

- Vegans do not consume animal products or by-products of animal products.

- They do not consume things such as eggs and milk.

- Real vegans, likewise, do not consume fish.

- Do not forget that bees are an animal, so vegans, likewise, can't consume royal jelly, honey and bee pollen supplements.

- There are, likewise, lots of concealed components to watch out for which have a tendency to make their way into food, including lard, gelatin and whey.

In case you are a brand-new vegan, incorporating all of these changes might appear overwhelming. However, after you have actually been eating and preparing the vegan way, you are going to be a pro.

WHAT THIS BOOK IS ABOUT

There's no question that a vegetarian diet plan, especially a vegan one, could be excellent for your health. Nevertheless, with the appeal of health food shops due to the truth that numerous are aiming to enhance their health, it's much easier than ever to take pleasure in a rewarding vegan diet plan. This guide is going to teach you how to do so.

- The fundamentals of how to prepare vegan food the proper way.

- A summary of common components utilized in vegan cooking.

- A list of hidden components to stay away from while consuming a vegan diet plan.

- Consists of information on stocking a complete vegan pantry so you could prepare vegan meals each day without any inconvenience.

- Will cover fundamental cooking methods required to make a range of pleasing meals.

- How to assemble a full vegan meal while getting the appropriate balance of minerals, vitamins and nutrients for your body.

- What to do if you have special dietary requirements like those who have high cholesterol or diabetes.

- Recipes so you could get going cooking immediately.

As you may see, there's a great deal of information to take in on how to take pleasure in a vegan diet plan. This guide is created to teach you whatever you have to understand.

CHAPTER 1: COMMON INGREDIENTS

As you understand, vegan cooking is cooking which is done without meat, eggs, fish or by-products of any of these things. So as to support a vegan way of life, additional care has to be taken to make certain that none of these components make it into the food.

We take specific things for granted, like utilizing eggs for baking. Well, eggs are not enabled throughout a vegan diet plan. And although the vegan way of life is going up in appeal, packaged vegan food is frequently difficult to come by. To fix this issue, numerous vegans decide to do their own cooking.

This chapter is going to concentrate on numerous various types of ingredients. Initially, we'll find out how to replace eggs and milk with things which are vegan-friendly. We'll cover information on other components which are utilized along with animal byproducts to keep an eye out for.

REPLACING EGGS

As much as we want to avoid utilizing eggs in our vegan dishes, it may be a hurdle. Actually, this is among the most challenging ingredients to substitute. Nevertheless, there are lots of alternatives to pick from that are going to do the job.

WHAT DO EGGS DO IN THE RECIPE?

In particular dishes, eggs are practically essential. They bind ingredients together. They could be utilized to make baked goods rise and they aid to make them fluffy and light. Eggs also help with structure formation, along with providing additional wetness. They are particularly helpful while baking but are necessary for specific tasty dishes too.

EGG REPLACEMENT OPTIONS

Here is a list of a few of the best egg replacement options out there. You could substitute the eggs in any dish utilizing these alternatives.

Pureed Bananas

Pureed bananas are one more reliable egg replacement. Simply put a ripe banana in the blender and pulse up until totally smooth and without lumps. A half of a regular-sized banana is the equivalent of a single egg.

The favorable aspect of utilizing bananas is that they are easily available. Nevertheless, bananas have a unique taste which will not work out in each dish. For instance, if you were attempting to make peanut butter cookies, the banana taste would change the taste.

Ground Flaxseeds

It is ideal to acquire the flaxseeds whole and keep them in the fridge. When it's time to utilize them, measure out 1 flaxseed tablespoon for each egg which you have to switch out. Then, crush it in a coffee mill or blender.

Move the flaxseeds to a bowl and include 3 tablespoons of water for every egg you have to switch out. Include the water gradually while whisking strongly. Whisk up until the mix takes on a gel-like quality.

Because flaxseeds are nutty-tasting, this egg replacement works ideally when making things such as muffins, whole-grain bread, and pancakes. You might wish to experiment to get a feel for the kinds of dishes you want this to be in.

Egg Replacement Product

There are plenty of egg replacement products out there that are created to be vegan-friendly. Take a look at the product packaging to ensure that it's vegan-friendly and that it does not consist of any meat byproducts.

These egg replacement powders receive mixed reviews. Certain folks like them, while others do not. They're certainly excellent and hassle-free to have on hand. When you get accustomed to cooking vegan, you'll begin to discover which foods taste ideally with it in it.

Given that there are a number of brands on the marketplace, it might take a bit to discover one which you're happiest with. When utilizing, simply follow the bundle guidelines. They generally can be found in powder form. In case you can't buy it at the health food shop, you could quickly get it online.

Try Tofu

Tofu is, likewise, another alternative you could have a go at if you have to discover a replacement product. You could attempt any type of tofu but this might take a bit of experimentation. Silken tofu appears to yield the ideal outcomes. You could, likewise, utilize unflavored soy yogurt in an identical percentage with comparable outcomes.

The good feature of tofu is that it mixes effectively with the majority of flavors. Flax seeds, for instance, have that special nutty taste. Tofu does not have a great deal of flavor by itself, specifically when coupled with more powerful ingredients. One more benefit is that it is commonly available in many locations, even in routine grocery stores.

To utilize, simply take the tofu and mix it up until smooth in the blender. A food processor, likewise, might work; however, it is necessary to make certain that there aren't any lumps and the texture is as smooth as it can be. To switch out one big egg, utilize a 1/4 cup of the blended mix.

You'll want to do a bit of experimenting to see which dishes work ideally with tofu as an egg replacement. All of it depends upon the types of dishes you attempt and your individual preferences.

Utilizing Flour and Other Leavening Agents

You could utilize pastes created from various sorts of flours and leavening agents to substitute the eggs. The advantage is that a lot of homes have these ingredients on hand. They, likewise, do not have a taste of their own such as flaxseeds and bananas do. They could mix into the batter relatively well.

It might take a bit of experimentation to get the percentages right. Here are certain alternatives:

- 1 tablespoon flour of any sort (try oat flour, wheat flour or soy flour) and 1 tablespoon water for every egg.

- 1 tablespoon flour, 1 tablespoon baking powder, 2 tablespoons water for every egg.

- 2 tablespoons water and 2 tablespoons corn starch mixed together to replace one egg.

Discovering the Right Egg Substitute

Once again, as you attempt these various combinations, you are going to get a feel for which egg substitutes work ideally for which dishes. As a recommendation, you might wish to begin with one of your preferred foods and have a go at various egg substitutes up until the texture and taste you want are reached.

For instance, if you wish to make a blueberry muffin batch, you could replace the eggs for any one of these substitution choices. Make a note of the taste. The following time you make it, have a go at another egg substitute. After attempting a number of them, consider which one was your favorite and stick to that. Pretty quickly, you'll have the ability to tell at a glimpse which egg replacement products work ideally for certain types of dishes.

REPLACING MILK

For a vegan, milk from any animal is additionally prohibited. It is also an extremely typical ingredient when cooking and baking. It is, likewise, a lot easier to substitute than eggs.

To substitute milk in recipes, simply replace any of these vegan alternatives. For instance, if the dish requires one cup of milk, utilize one cup of soy milk rather. Here are certain milk alternatives:

- Soy milk

Soy milk tends to be in a range of flavors and is available readily. Flavors consist of chocolate, vanilla, and even egg nog. Certain brands are creamier and thicker than others. You might want to do some experimenting before you discover the brands you like the most. Unless it has a unique flavoring, soy milk is relatively neutral and mixes well in recipes. Soy milk is additionally abundant in protein.

- Nut milk

Nut milk drinks like hazelnut milk and almond milk are likewise options. Unlike soy milk, nut milk has a unique taste and might not work well in each dish. There are unsweetened and sweetened varieties too.

- Rice milk

Rice milk provides an excellent option to replace milk in dishes. It is additionally extremely moderate tasting and blends effectively in recipes. Anyhow, it is essential to bear in mind that rice milk normally does not consist of a great deal of protein, which means you may have to make up for that throughout the day.

As you end up being knowledgeable about the various flavors of these milk replacement products, you'll begin to get a feel for which recipes are going to taste ideally with them.

REPLACING BUTTERMILK IN RECIPES

Buttermilk is, likewise, an essential ingredient utilized in a number of various dishes. For a vegan, utilizing standard buttermilk is difficult, given that it is an animal product. Buttermilk is just regular milk which has actually been cultured, and that indicates that it has some excellent bacteria in it, just like yogurt.

Fortunately, you could quickly make your own. The procedure is the following. It yields one cup of vegan-friendly "buttermilk."

1. Measure a single cup of soy milk in a measuring cup.

2. Measure out the identical quantity in soy milk.

3. Add 1 tablespoon of lemon juice or vinegar and mix.

4. Allow it sit for approximately fifteen minutes prior to utilizing it.

Soy milk works ideally. Nut milk and rice milk aren't good choices. The chemistry of soy milk is much more appropriate.

REPLACING LARD AND BUTTER

Butter is one more crucial ingredient which a great deal of recipes require. There are a number of various things you may do so as to substitute it:

- Vegetable oil

If the recipe requires melted, or perhaps strong, butter, you can think about utilizing vegetable oil rather. This, nevertheless, might change the recipe texture a bit, so you are going to most likely have to experiment.

- Shortening.

If you truly require a solid fat to utilize in recipes, you could utilize vegan-friendly shortening. This is loaded with trans fats, nevertheless. So, utilizing it in small amounts is best. Shortening isn't great for you whatsoever! You could additionally discover butter-flavored shortening where a butter flavor is needed.

- Margarine.

This is one more option which could substitute butter or other solid fats, specifically if you desire something with a buttery flavor. Nevertheless, margarine is additionally high in trans-fatty acids. Look for transfat-free products, however, even those might consist of trace quantities of trans fats.

- Minimizing fat.

You could additionally minimize fat with fruit purees. For instance, if the dish requires 1 cup of butter, you could attempt utilizing 1/2 cup vegan margarine or shortening and 1/2 cup apple sauce. Other fruit purees you could utilize consists of banana puree and plum puree. You might have the ability to discover fruit puree fat replacement items in the shop. Simply make certain they are vegan-friendly and that you follow the guidelines for making an appropriate substitution. You might, likewise, wish to try replacing all the fat in the dish with fruit. Nevertheless, this might change the texture excessively.

Constantly ensure that the butter replacement products are utilized in small amounts. A diet plan which is high in fats and trans fats is not a healthy diet plan. If you definitely require them, simply utilize them occasionally.

COMMON INGREDIENTS

Vegan cooking is definitely an art. As shown in the prior part, ingredients like milk, eggs, buttermilk, and butter are nearly essential for certain dishes. However, as we explored, the substitutions are more than sufficient. With that stated, there are a great deal of ingredients which a great deal of vegan chefs find vital. Here's a rundown of a few of the most frequent.

SOY PRODUCTS

Soy is most likely the most versatile plant out there, particularly when it pertains to making protein-rich and healthy vegan meals. Here is a list of a few of the soy items which are out there:

- Soy milk

This is readily available and could be discovered in a number of various flavors, like chocolate and vanilla.

- Tofu.

Tofu can be found in various levels of firmness, like extra soft or firm.

- Tempeh.

Tempeh is a fermented product that has a meaty, hearty texture which could be utilized in stir fries and other meals.

- Ground Meat replacement.

This soy option is a staple to certain people, due to the fact that you can make meals like vegan chili and Spaghetti Bolognese.

- Soy yogurt.

Consists of active cultures similar to regular yogurt and can be found in a range of flavors.

- Miso.

Miso is a fermented salty paste which is created from soy and is utilized as a prominent, enzyme-rich soup base.

- Soy Sauce and Tamari.

Both condiments are created from soy.

- Edamame.

These are the fresh soybeans and are exceptional on their own or in stir fries.

- Soy cheese

Soy cheese even melts and has a comparable texture as actual cheese.

- Soy sausage, hamburger patties and hot dogs

Vegans could delight in hotdogs, breakfast sausage and even hamburger patties.

- Soy "chicken."

They are available in plenty of types like nuggets, patties and so on.

- Soy protein powder.

Soy protein provides an excellent method to increase your everyday protein consumption. You could place a scoop in your morning smoothie, or include it to dishes like bread and pancakes.

- Soy flour.

This is, likewise, an important product, especially for baking.

There are a great deal of soy products out there and this is not a comprehensive list. It simply shows the versatility of the food product. Try to find soy products which are utilized from non-genetically modified soybeans.

However, soy foods have their critics. Some just like to utilize them in their standard forms like tempeh, tofu, edamame, miso and tamari. Processed soy product opponents are wary of the reality that they are developed to taste like milk or meat products which to them, defeats the purpose veganism. Plus, these foods have a tendency to be extremely processed and that does not always make them healthier. Whether you choose to utilize them is a choice that you need to make after you weigh the benefits and drawbacks.

WHOLE GRAINS.

There are a lot of various types of whole grains, it is worth experimenting. Grains are abundant in minerals, vitamins, fiber, and other essential nutrients. They even have protein, specifically quinoa-- an ancient grain which is particularly protein-rich. Here are certain whole grain products to test out:

- Buckwheat.

- Rye.

- Wheat products.

- Quinoa.

- Brown rice.

- Pasta.

- Oats.

These could be ground into flour or utilized whole. They ought to form the foundation of a healthy vegan diet.

SEEDS AND NUTS

These are another vital part of a healthy vegan diet. They are abundant in minerals and vitamins in addition to essential nutrients such as healthy fats. Here's a list of some seeds and nuts to try out:

- Walnuts.

- Hazelnuts (filberts).

- Sunflower seeds.

- Pecans.

- Pumpkin seeds.

- Almonds.

- Sesame seeds.

- Cashews.

- Poppy seeds.

- Hemp seeds.

- Flax seeds.

You could add them in recipes and additionally consume them by themselves as a treat.

LEGUMES.

Legumes are an important protein source to a vegan, particularly when coupled with whole grains. They have to be combined in this manner so that they can form a complete protein. When this is one of your primary sources of protein, it is necessary to bear in mind to combine it.

Here are certain instances. This list is in no way extensive:

- Lentils.

- Chickpeas (garbanzo beans).

- Kidney beans.

- Cannelloni beans.

- Black beans.

- Black eyed peas.

- Northern beans.

- Split peas.

You could discover legumes in dried form, canned and ground into flour. The dried form has to be drenched overnight if you want to soften it. The canned form is simple to utilize and terrific to have on hand. The flour is a well-known ingredient in baked foods and tasty cooking.

VEGETABLES AND FRUITS.

Essential for good health, vegetables and fruits include variety and color to your meals. As a vegan, your whole diet plan is going to be plant-based, so you have to obtain your minerals, vitamins and nutrients from things such as vegetables and fruits.

Search for organic fruit and vegetables whenever you can that makes them even healthier. Organic food is additionally much better for the environment. Seasonal, local produce is additionally ideal due to the fact that it aids to support your regional economy and tastes a great deal fresher.

CANNED AND PACKAGED FOODS.

As the vegan diet plan boosts in appeal, so does the accessibility of packaged, vegan-friendly foods. Here is a list of a few of the things you could discover.

- Bread.

- Baked goods.

- Desserts.

- Vegan chocolate.

- Snacks.

- Canned goods.

- Breakfast foods and cereals.

- Drinks.

- And so on.

The fantastic thing is that you do not even have to go to an organic food shop to discover a great deal of these items. Yes, organic food shops have a great deal of vegan options, however, you could even discover vegan products in your routine grocery store.

Print it out so that you could discover the things which you require when you go to the shop. We'll take a look at a few of these products in greater detail as we discuss how to stock a total vegan pantry.

INGREDIENTS TO WATCH OUT FOR

As discussed in a previous part, there are frequently concealed ingredients in foods which are animal byproducts. A real vegan is going to take the additional step required to find out what these ingredients are.

In case

 it is a packaged food and it is labeled as vegan-friendly, you could be relatively positive that the food does not have these ingredients in it. However, it is still an excellent idea to examine.

Up next is an ingredient list to keep an eye out for. There are 2 types of ingredients-- those that are plainly from animal products, and those which might be from plant-derived or animal products.

In the 2nd classification, the only way to truly find things out is by calling the maker of the food product. And if they can not answer your question, think about not purchasing their item simply to be safe.

INGREDIENTS FROM ANIMALS.

These ingredients are relatively frequent in foods, so unless an item is labeled as vegan, you need to truly inspect the ingredient list to ensure they aren't included.

- Albumin - comes from egg whites.

- Milk products - includes whey protein powder, lactose, lactase, and things such as dried milk and milk.

- Calcium Caseinate-- a relatively frequent additive.

Calcium Stearate - yet another additive

Suet - a kind of animal fat

Tallow - an animal fat product created from suet

Bee products - this consists of royal jelly, honey, propolis, and bee pollen

Carmine - a food additive which originates from pests

Lard - a kind of animal fat

Casein - the protein found in cheese

Gelatin - from animals, a well-known item discovered specifically in desserts and jellies.

Other typical concealed ingredients from animals consist of:

Isinglass.

Cochineal.

Oleic acid.

Palmitic acid.

Muriatic acid.

Pepsin.

Pancreatin.

The majority of the above ingredients are usually utilized as food additives. They have various functions, based upon the food that it is going to go on.

INGREDIENTS THAT MAY BE FROM ANIMALS

These ingredients serve various functions in the food that they remain in. Some are seen as additives. Others emulsify foods and offer additional fats. Nevertheless, even if it seems like an animal ingredient, it doesn't mean it is. They may be artificially produced or come from plants. You'll want to check it out.

The ingredients consist of:

Fatty acid.

Emulsifying agents.

Adipic acid.

Glyceride.

Capric acid.

Glycerol.

Lactic acid.

Monoglyceride.

Magnesium stearate.

Anything noted as a natural flavoring.

Disodium inosinate.

Clarifying agents.

Glyceride.

Glycerol.

Diglyceride.

Stearic acid.

Polysorbate.

Sodium stearoyl lactylate.

Yes, a few of those ingredients are difficult to pronounce. Some of them don't even sound like food! They all have their parts in the foods which we consume daily, even foods which we don't take into consideration. The bottom line is that if you wish to live a really vegan lifestyle, it is worth the additional step to follow up and identify if your favorite foods utilize the animal versions of these ingredients.

Nevertheless, it is necessary to comprehend that the ingredients pointed out in this part could be discovered in nearly everything. If you attempt to focus excessively on it, it might get too overwhelming. It is necessary to discover an excellent balance between wishing to be a meticulous vegan and living a satisfying life. If things go too far, it might impact your health in an unfavorable way from the tension.

Being a vegan is absolutely a lifestyle dedication. Learning more about the foods you have to consume, how to make vegan-friendly alternatives while cooking and baking, and all about the ingredients you might wish to stay away from are all required parts of accepting the vegan lifestyle.

CHAPTER 2: THE VEGAN PANTRY

Establishing your pantry is an important step to being able to make meals on a whim. For individuals who have actually been vegetarians their whole lives, establishing the pantry is not going to be a struggle. Nevertheless, if you've simply recently converted to a vegan, you'll most likely want to go back to square one. You might have certain ingredients on hand, however, the majority of your pantry might not be vegan-friendly.

Naturally, this list is not going to consist of perishable products like vegetables and fruits. Nevertheless, even some perishable products, like particular brands of tofu, rice milk, almond milk, soy milk, etc. could be kept on the shelves due to the special packaging.

STEP ONE

The initial step to developing a vegan pantry is to take stock of what you have. This step is primarily for those who have simply ended up being vegans. Nevertheless, if you have been vegan for some time, you are going to additionally gain from this. The objective is to go through and consider all that you have and figure out if it supports the vegan way of life.

You might additionally wish to take a look at the ingredients lists of all your packaged foods to identify if any of the concealed ingredients noted in the previous chapter exist. Even if you have actually been vegan for some time, you might still discover certain foods within your pantry that shouldn't be there.

If you do discover a great deal of foods to do away with and they have actually not been opened, do not toss them away. Give them away to a nearby food pantry. Even if you are not going to eat them does not indicate that somebody is not going to gain from them and value having something to eat.

STEP TWO

It isn't completely required to have a big pantry filled with lots of components and packaged foods. All you have to do is sit and consider the things which are actually crucial to you. If you do not bake that frequently, for instance, don't bother purchasing baking supplies up until you actually require them. If you are the kind of individual who enjoys cereal and has a couple of bowls a day, you might wish to keep packages of nut milk, rice milk, soy milk and extra cereal in your pantry so you do not have to go to the shop constantly.

As soon as you figure out what you require and what your eating choices are, then you could begin purchasing things to place in your pantry. If you do not take the additional time to consider what you require, you'll wind up buying things you will not eat. Then, the food is going to go to waste. Simply stock the fundamentals and if you require other things, you could purchase them as you go along.

STEP THREE

It could be costly to stock your pantry simultaneously. There are specific ingredients which you might require occasionally, like a tomato sauce and other items. It isn't essential to purchase a few of these extras in the beginning. You could include to your pantry slowly as you go shopping or as you recognize you require them.

Generally, it is good to have the ingredients nearby to make a couple of basic meals like soups, pasta meals and legume and grain dinners like beans and rice. Consider the sorts of foods you like to buy and eat the additional ingredients to have within your reach.

In you are on a strict budget, you could take care of these items as you go along. Plan your meals ahead of time and draw up a shopping list. You could purchase these additionals at the start of the week and store them as you purchase them.

EXAMPLE

Despite the fact that pantries might vary from home to home, it is going to be useful to see a sample pantry. You could utilize this as a beginning point while attempting to determine how to stock yours, or you could simply take this list to the shop and begin shopping! It's up to you.

It might aid to consider your pantry in regards to classifications like breakfast items, treats, and so on. Here's a rough list:

BREAKFAST ITEMS

- Whole-grain hot cereals like cream of wheat or oatmeal

- Cold cereals to eat with nut milk, soy milk, or rice milk

- Vegan-friendly pancake blends

- Vegan baked goods like muffins

SNACKS

- A range of healthy snack items like granola bars

- Vegan treats like cakes and cookies

- Crackers and other baked items

MISC. ITEMS

- Nut milk, rice milk, soy milk, , and tofu in unique packaging to aid it store in the kitchen and remain fresh longer

- Soup blends, canned soups and other boxed meal items like vegan macaroni and cheese

- Seeds and nuts like almonds, sunflower seeds, sesame seeds and pecans.

- Pasta-- search for whole wheat varieties

- Items such as spaghetti sauce, pickles, capers, salad dressings, additional ketchup, and so on.

GRAIN PRODUCTS.

These are simply a couple of instances. Purchase things which are in accordance with your preferences.

- Buckwheat flour.

- Whole wheat rice.

- Wheat flour.

- Quinoa.

DRESSINGS.

- One vegetable oil to cook with.

- At least one type of tasty oil like roasted sesame oil or cold-pressed olive oil.

- Tamara and/ or soy sauce.

- Vinegar-- you could keep a number of kinds on hand like rice wine, balsamic, and red wine vinegar.

- Pepper, salt, spices and herbs.

BAKING PRODUCTS

- Leavening agents like baking powder, yeast, and baking soda

- Vegan-friendly egg replacement

- Various types of flours

- Sugars and other sweetener items like rice syrup and maple syrup.

This list is simply created to be a jumping-off point. It is nearly impossible to come up with a blanket list due to the fact that individuals' food preferences differ considerably. The strategy many people like to use is to buy things one at a time as you require them.

Keep in mind to look at the ingredients, particularly when you are purchasing packaged food. As we've explored, there are typically concealed ingredients which are not vegan-friendly where you would least expect them.

CHAPTER 3: VEGAN COOKING FUNDAMENTALS

So, we have actually spent a long time considering a few of the frequent ingredients which are generally included in vegan foods. We have actually found out how to stock the pantry and additionally discover concealed ingredients in foods which vegans should not eat.

The next action is to, in fact, find out how to cook.

If you currently know how to cook, you could bypass this chapter. However, I would advise reading it anyway due to the fact that there may be things in here you do not already understand. To get the correct instruction, you truly ought to cook with somebody who understands what they are doing.

Or even better, you could take a few cooking classes. Search around your location to see if you can discover any vegan cooking classes which could offer you an excellent introduction to a few of the methods.

Although we are going to go over the methods you have to understand how to assemble a range of foods within this chapter, it could be enjoyable learning in a group environment.

Here is a fundamental list of a few of the methods you require:

- Establishing your kitchen area
- How to follow a recipe
- Fundamental cooking techniques

Individuals might spend a lifetime finding out how to cook and not even scratch the surface. So, we'll discuss a few of the fundamental techniques. If you wish to discover more, you ought to, most likely, think about registering for a class.

SETTING UP YOUR KITCHEN

As discussed in the prior chapter, stocking your pantry is a crucial bit of the vegan cooking puzzle. The other is to have a fully equipped kitchen area to cook an assortment of dishes.

Now, there are 2 kinds of chefs out there. Those who like to utilize a great deal of gadgets and those who do not. A lot of home cooks have a tendency to fall someplace in between.

Here's a list of a few of the fundamental kitchen products you want to have in order to be able to make a number of recipes. If you stumble upon something that you wish to make that requires specialized equipment, you could either think about purchasing it or making a substitution.

- A great set of knives which consist of a chef's knife and bread knife. Unless they are serrated, ensure you maintain them sharp. You'll additionally want a big cutting board.

- An electric mixer. If you do a great deal of baking, you might wish to discover an upright mixer which rests on your countertop.

- Numerous utensils like a pair of durable thongs, wooden spoons, a sieve, rubber spatulas, and a strong wire whisk.

- A small toaster, microwave and an oven.

- A blender and/or a food processor.

- Optional, however great to have nearby-- a submersion mixer, ice cream maker, crockpot, a bread maker in case you need freshly baked bread.

- A great assortment of pans, pots, and blending bowls.

Certain individuals make the blunder of purchasing everything simultaneously. This is a mistake, particularly if you're brand-new to cooking. You'll begin to comprehend your individual style.

HOW TO FOLLOW RECIPES

Learning how to follow recipes is an extremely crucial ability in discovering how to cook. The majority of recipes are quite simple. Nevertheless, it is simple to take them for granted up until something is going wrong. There are numerous handwritten recipes out there which exclude important ingredients without meaning to. If you discover a recipe such as this, having an excellent understanding of how recipes work could aid you decipher the ingredient which is missing.

If you are simply finding out how to cook, you are going to be following recipes constantly. Nevertheless, as you get comfier in the kitchen area, you'll slowly begin to lose your reliance on them.

After you follow a couple of recipes, you could begin to write your own original meals down. Simply keep in mind to note the ingredients in the order that they are going to show up in the directions. This makes the recipe simpler to follow.

COOKING TECHNIQUES

After you established your kitchen area and you make certain you comprehend how to follow recipes, the next action is to find out certain fundamental cooking techniques. Here is a short list of a few of the things you'll want to do in order to cook.

DISCOVER HOW TO UTILIZE YOUR KNIVES

There is a wrong and right way to slice. Many folks do not think much about it. Nevertheless, the incorrect method can get you hurt and additionally make you ineffective. In order to learn, you'll wish to work with an expert. Constantly make certain your knives are sharp, as well. It's really more unsafe if they're dull.

If you do not wish to take cooking classes in order to learn appropriate slicing techniques, you might always see a cooking show on tv and imitate what they do.

It is necessary to have a premium chef's knife on hand. When cooking specific things, like soups and salads, the majority of your time is spent slicing. If you find out how to be efficient, you could save a great deal of time.

HEATING, BOILING AND SIMMERING

These are 3 really fundamental cooking techniques for the stove top. Boiling is when you generally set the heat on high and wait for the whole thing to bubble. When you heat something, you allow it to get hot but not boiling hot. When you simmer something, you place it on low heat for a long amount of time. Things such as stews and soups, for instance, are usually simmered.

BAKING AND BROILING

The terms broiling and baking are not identical. Nevertheless, certain things that could be baked could additionally be broiled and vice versa. Baking occurs at a lower heat than broiling. Classic things which are baked consist of cookies, bread, cakes, and mouthwatering meals like roasted veggies and vegetarian lasagna. Things such as vegetarian lasagna, for instance, could likewise be broiled.

A lot of ovens are equipped with a broiler. Nevertheless, everyone is different. You'll want to read your handbook so as to find out how to operate yours.

HOW TO UTILIZE ALL OF YOUR APPLIANCES

One more essential step to developing vegan dishes is to ensure you comprehend how to utilize all of your appliances. For instance, you might not know it, but your microwave might additionally have a convection oven setting. You might not recognize what it's capable of up until you check out the manual.

You'll have the ability to make modifications in recipes based upon how your appliances work. For instance, if the directions state to beat something on high for 2 minutes, your mixer might take more if the "high" setting is not as effective as the mixer utilized to evaluate and write the initial recipe.

COMMON COOKING TERMS AND WHAT THEY MEAN

When you get familiarized with your kitchen area and begin following some recipes, you might discover some terms which you do not understand what to do with. Here are certain typical ones you might come across:

- Mashing.

You could either mash with a masher tool or a fork. Some individuals choose to whip things which are usually mashed like squash or potatoes.

- Whip.

You could utilize an upright mixer, a hand mixer or a wire whisk to whip almost everything.

- Crush.

You could crush things with the rear of your knife, the bottom of a glass, or other heavy things. There are special kitchen area gizmos utilized for crushing.

- Grate.

Graters are available in various forms. Simply choose. If you have to grate lemon peel or an orange peel, a little handheld grater is best.

- Knife techniques.

There are numerous various sorts of knife techniques you could do involving chop, julienne (match stick sized pieces), crush, and slice.

- Blend.

Based upon what you are mixing, you have 3 options-- a regular blender, a handheld submersion blender that functions ideally for soups, and a food processor. The tool you utilize is going to depend upon the dish.

- Puree.

When a recipe instructs you to puree a thing, you could do it in little batches in the standard blender, utilize a submersion blender, or utilize the food processor.

This is simply a summary of a few of the methods you are going to experience. An excellent, thorough cookbook is going to aid you to specify any other terms you have to understand. Or, you could look on the web.

CHAPTER 4: A COMPLETE MEAL

Even if somebody is a vegan does not suggest they are going to be naturally healthy and thin. This is due to the fact that it is still feasible to have too many calories as a vegan, regardless of the wealth of nutrient-dense foods to pick from. Every effort has to be undertaken to develop well-balanced meals.

This could be a hurdle, particularly if you are first beginning as a vegan. One reason for this is since specific minerals and vitamins, like Iron and Vitamin B12, are more quickly discovered in meat products. Additionally, Iron is more readily absorbed in the body when coupled with meat.

CONSIDERATIONS

This part is going to cover a few of the obstacles vegans deal with when putting meals together. It is created to aid you create healthy and well-balanced meal combinations which are going to leave you healthy and lively. If you wish to drop weight or remain thin, simply keep in mind not to eat too many calories in addition.

GETTING AMPLE PROTEIN

Individuals who eat meat take getting ample protein for granted. All they have to do is take in dairy products and a serving or 2 of fish or meat a day in order to do it. However, vegans have to get their protein from plant sources. Thankfully, there are things in the plant realm which are still abundant in protein:

- Soy products

- Seeds, nuts, nut butter and nut milk.

- Grains, particularly quinoa

- Legumes like kidney beans. Keep in mind to eat a serving of grain at the identical meal.

You might additionally wish to consume a serving or 2 of protein drink daily. Simply ensure the packaging shows that it is vegan-friendly. A prominent ingredient in the majority of protein powders is whey, and that is from milk and ought to be avoided.

EATING AMPLE IRON

For ladies, getting ample iron is enough of a hurdle. For a vegan, it's even harder and lots of vegans wind up with iron shortages. On the advice of your physician, you might wish to take an iron supplement. You could discover vegan-friendly, plant-based iron supplements at the organic food shop. Additionally, eat these foods:

- Green beans.
- Spinach.
- Wheat germ.
- Brewer's yeast (a supplement).
- Lima beans.
- Cooking in a cast-iron skillet.
- Dried fruit like prunes and raisins.
- Blackstrap molasses (utilize in baking or take as a supplement).

If you want to make plant protein more absorbable, combine it with a vitamin C abundant food, drink, or supplement. For instance, you could have a little glass of orange with a meal which has a great deal of iron.

FOODS ABUNDANT IN B-VITAMINS

Vegans get enough of the majority of the B Vitamins since grains are a great source. Nevertheless, Vitamin B 12 is a bit harder. The only option for this is to supplement it with a vegan-friendly variation of B 12, which is frequently artificial. Some drinks and cereals consist of B 12.

GETTING AMPLE CALCIUM

Thanks to fortification, it is simpler than ever for a vegan to obtain their calcium. Here are certain foods to have:

- Nut milk, soy milk and rice milk are typically fortified with calcium. Ensure the product is vegan-friendly and comprises of a great quantity of calcium.

- Nuts like almonds and hazelnuts are additionally a great calcium source.

- Leafy green veggies and other veggies like collard greens, bok choy, turnip greens, and okra are additionally abundant in calcium.

When preparing the veggies, attempt not to boil them unless you drink the water. A great deal of the calcium leaves the food throughout the cooking procedure and goes into the water.

GETTING IT RIGHT

If you have actually been a vegan for some time, you might currently have the hang of this. If not, you might wish to plan a few of your meals out ahead of time up until you get the hang of it. Even if you have actually been a vegan for some time, it's an excellent idea to take a step back and prepare a few meals occasionally. Not just is this going to help make sure that you get the nutrients you require, but it aids to create variety since you could plan meals around brand-new ingredients.

Besides preparing meals, you could additionally have a food journal. In it, monitor what you eat, how you cooked it, whether you like it, and if you would alter anything. It's additionally a great method to see if you are obtaining the appropriate nutrients. You do not need to evaluate it too intensely. You could simply glance at it to ensure you're getting what you require.

It's a great idea to take a multivitamin supplement along with consuming a healthy diet plan. This is going to ensure your body has what it requires to maintain you healthy.

VEGAN-FRIENDLY ETHNIC CUISINE

There are numerous ethnic cuisines which are mainly vegetarian. As a result, they have a great deal of delicious vegan meals which you could take pleasure in. This provides your diet with much-needed variety.

Here is a short list of a few of the foods out there. The majority of these also have meat meals, but their vegetarian choices are really delicious.

- Indian.

There are lots of vegetable-based and grain options.

- Chinese.

The Buddhist monks consume a largely vegetarian diet plan.

- French.

Fresh vegetables and fruits form the centerpiece of this Mediterranean cuisine.

- Italian.

Italian food concentrates on fresh vegetables and fruits

- Korean.

Great deal of veggies and rice are consumed daily.

- Thai.

Similar to standard produce based Chinese food, Thai likewise packs some heat.

- Vietnamese.

Another Asian food which utilizes a great deal of plant-based foods.

- Greek.

One more Mediterranean region cuisine which features a great deal of fresh produce.

This list is in no way extensive. For instance, Mediterranean cuisine, generally, is vegan-friendly due to the fact that there are a great deal of dishes which concentrate on plant-based foods. There are a great deal of countries which comprise that region consisting of France, Greece, Italy, Morocco, Spain, and Algeria.

Asian cuisine, generally, has a great deal of dishes which are made mainly from plant-based foods. Even if something such as a stir fry requires some meat, you could quickly leave it out without harming the flavors.

CHAPTER 5: SPECIAL CONSIDERATIONS.

The vegan diet plan is a perfect one for establishing health. As pointed out in a previous chapter, nevertheless, it is still feasible for there to be obese vegans due to the fact that all you have to do is take in too many calories. You could, likewise, be unhealthy as a vegan by not obtaining enough of the appropriate nutrients. Nevertheless, those issues could be quickly repaired by cutting calories and producing much better, more comprehensive meals.

Nevertheless, certain individuals have larger health issues to think about. Some might be utilizing the vegan diet plan to aid them restore their health. Others picked to end up being vegans for other reasons and it just so occurs they have health issues like diabetes.

Here is a list of certain typical health conditions and how to change the vegan diet to accommodate it. Keep in mind that the vegan diet is a healthy diet plan, to start, so it makes these changes a great deal simpler.

DIABETES

There are 2 types of diabetes-- Type 1, which individuals are born with, and Type 2, which comes later on in life. The vegan diet plan, particularly a low-fat one, is particularly helpful for individuals who have Type 2 diabetes. Nevertheless, Type 1 victims could additionally benefit.

If you adhere to low-fat foods, nuts, whole grains, seeds, legumes, and lots of vegetables and fruits, it is going to aid to manage your condition naturally. Additionally, ensure to take the medication you ought to. When your body can't create insulin or does not produce enough, there's no other method for your body to obtain it except for the medication.

CIRCULATORY DISEASES

Circulatory system diseases, like hypertension, high cholesterol, and generalized heart disease, all gain from the vegan diet plan naturally. This is since it is low in cholesterol and fat. Likewise, if you have hypertension, you could take an additional step and make certain that you do not consume excessive amount of salt.

This is one more instance where abiding by the vegan diet plan benefits your health and could aid with these health issues.

LOW-FAT DIET

The vegan diet plan is naturally low in fat. As a matter of fact, since you are not taking in any meat items, it is high in the useful fats and low in saturated fats that originate from nuts, avocado and seeds, and different vegetable oils.

Nevertheless, there are certain things to remember. Initially, keep away from trans fats. In numerous ways, these are even worse for you than saturated fats. Likewise, you might require a tiny amount of saturated fat in your diet plan. You could get what you require by consuming coconut every once in a while. You could additionally cook with coconut oil, that might take the place of lard or butter.

LOW SUGAR COOKING

If you follow the vegan diet plan as it should be followed, the vegan diet plan is naturally low in sugar. Nevertheless, much like with any way of life, there is the chance that you can overdo it. Yes, your body requires some sugar. You could obtain it naturally from dried and fresh fruits along with sugar cane, maple syrup or rice syrup.

Nevertheless, there are, likewise, baked goods and other sugary possibilities (like vegan-friendly chocolate) which could end up being just as addicting as their non-vegan equivalents. Moderation is the key. If you wish to follow a low sugar diet plan, train your body to take pleasure in sugar in its natural state when it's present in fruit and not to delight in baked foods.

LOW SODIUM COOKING

Individuals who follow the vegan diet plan are just as susceptible to taking in excessive salt as anybody else. The vegan diet plan is low in sodium. However, grab the salt shaker frequently, and this might adversely impact your health.

Processed and packaged foods exist no matter if you are a vegan or not. So does the salt shaker. Stay away from it, particularly if you tend to retain water or if you have hypertension.

GLUTEN-FREE COOKING

At first glance, it might look like a hurdle to do away with gluten on a vegan diet plan. Nevertheless, it is still extremely feasible. If you have to stay away from gluten, here is a short list of a few of the grains to stay away from:

- Barley.

- Oats.

- Wheat.

- Kamut.

- Rye.

- Spelt.

Nevertheless, there are still a lot of starches and grains which you could consume.

- Rice, particularly brown rice.

- Corn.

- Quinoa.

- Potatoes.

- Millet.

Simply follow the vegan diet plan as you usually would, however, just stick to those grains which do not produce gluten.

As you could see, you could quickly adjust to the vegan diet plan to assist with a variety of health issues.

CHAPTER 6: RECIPES.

Now, it's time to put all of it together and attempt some brand-new recipes. This part offers you a sampling of a few of the recipes you could whip up a vegan diet plan. Do not hesitate to adjust and alter them as you choose. People's tastes vary and you might, likewise, wish to alter things around based upon your state of mind or what you have on hand.

Have a cooking journal so you could monitor what you liked and didn't like about a prticular recipe. That way, if you make something you enjoy, you could replicate it. If you didn't quite like it, you could make changes the following time.

APPETIZERS

Bruschetta

A traditional Italian meal which works as a treat or appetizer. This is naturally vegan.

Ingredients:

1/4 cup scallions, sliced.

1 clove garlic, minced.

1 big tomato, diced.

Olive oil.

6 pieces fresh, whole grain bakery bread.

1 tablespoon dried basil.

Directions:

Preheat oven to 350 degrees. In a little blending bowl, combine first 4 ingredients. Spray nonstick cooking spray over a baking sheet and arrange sliced bread on sheet. Spoon tomato mixture equally over all 4 pieces. Drizzle with olive oil. Bake for approximately 15 minutes, or up until bread is toasted.

Black Olive Hummus

Hummus is a traditional vegetarian food that is high in protein and low in fat. Spread on vegan crackers, whole grain or serve with bread.

Ingredients:

1 15 oz can prepared chickpeas, washed and drained

1/3 cup fresh lemon juice

1 tablespoon water

1/4 cup pitted black olives, diced

Directions:

Mix all of the ingredients in a blender or food processor and pulse up until it is creamy. Move it to a serving dish and offer with bread, crackers or whole-grain pita wedges.

SOUPS

Greek-Style Chickpea Soup

This is an instance of a hearty Greek meal which is vegan-friendly. Offer with pieces of fresh, salad and a whole grain bread.

Ingredients:

3 15 ounce cans of chickpeas, washed and drained

1 teaspoon dried rosemary

1 big onion, sliced

3 tablespoons fresh, sliced parsley

1 teaspoon sea salt

1 can crushed tomatoes (with juice).

4 cloves garlic, sliced fine

3 cups water.

Pepper and salt to taste.

2 tablespoons olive oil.

Directions:

Place all of the ingredients in a big pot. Bring to a boil, and after that, simmer on low temperature for an hour up until flavors are well mixed. You are able to, likewise, cook it in a crock pot on the low setting for 4-6 hours.

Classic Minestrone Soup

This is an all-time favorite. The great feature of it is that you could utilize whichever veggies you have nearby. This recipe could get you started.

Ingredients:

2 big carrots, sliced and peeled.

1 medium onion, sliced.

3 celery stalks, sliced.

2 cloves garlic, minced.

1 cup broccoli florets.

1 cup spinach leaves.

2 zucchini, sliced.

1 can crushed tomatoes.

8 cups water.

1 cup canned kidney beans, washed.

1 cup little pasta like orzo.

Fresh sliced parsley for a garnish.

Salt and pepper to taste.

Directions:

Mix all of the ingredients other than the pasta in a soup pot. Bring to a boil and after that simmer for at least an hour up until the veggies are soft. Include pasta throughout the last fifteen minutes of cooking and cook for 8 to 10 minutes. You could additionally cook the soup in the crock pot. Simply include all of the ingredients at the same time.

SALADS

Vegan Cesar Salad

The Cesar salad is timeless, but the dressing is certainly not vegan-friendly. This recipe alters that.

Dressing Ingredients:

1/2 cup brewer's yeast

1/2 cup vegan mayo

Juice of 1 lemon

2 teaspoons cracked pepper

Salad Ingredients:

1 cup sliced black olives

4 cups torn romaine lettuce leaves

3 tablespoons grated soy parmesan.

Directions:

At the bottom of a big salad bowl, blend all of the salad dressing ingredients together. Toss in the romaine lettuce up until dressing is properly covered. Top with parmesan cheese and black olives and serve.

Traditional Salad

The traditional salad is, naturally, vegan-friendly. Simply pick the veggies which you desire and the dressing which you desire, as long as it is vegan. You could create your own vegan dressings, as well. Vinaigrettes are particularly easy since all they need is equal parts of oil and vinegar blended together. You could additionally include pepper, salt and spices to taste.

Salads are nice since you could utilize whatever you have in the house. Have your refrigerator well equipped with vegetables and fruit and you could create a healthy salad whenever you desire.

MAIN COURSES

Vegan Lentil Tacos

Lentils make a good replacement for the standard beef which typically goes in tacos.

Ingredients:

1 cup dried, brown lentils

1 packet taco spices mix (vegan).

1 8 ounce can of tomato sauce

Shredded romaine lettuce.

Corn tortillas or taco shells.

Cucumber pieces.

Soy sour cream.

Sliced, fresh tomatoes.

Salsa.

Guacamole.

Directions:

Soak the lentils in a big bowl up until soft, for around an hour. Move to a saucepan and combine with taco spices and tomato sauce. Include around 1/4 cup of water. Simmer on low up until heated up through. Spoon into tortillas or taco shells and top with things such as sour cream, lettuce, salsa, tomato and cucumber.

Healthy Vegetable Casserole

Casseroles are one more healthy supper choice for vegans. The good aspect of them is when you have the recipe down pat, you could create a lot of them.

Ingredients:

1 cup cooked brown rice.

1 8 ounce can of tomato soup.

1 8 ounce can legumes like kidney beans or chickpeas.

4 cups veggies of choice-- have a go at mushrooms, zucchini, celery, carrots, tomatoes, eggplant, onions, leeks, garlic, potatoes

Directions:

Spray a medium casserole meal with nonstick cooking spray. Layer with brown rice. Include veggies on top of the rice. You could blend the veggies together, select one kind of veggie, or layer different kinds-- it depends on you. Pour soup over veggies. Cover and bake at 350 degrees for approximately 40 minutes.

SIDE DISHES

When it pertains to side dishes, there are a great deal of choices for you. Here is a list of certain ideas:

- Cover a baking sheet with veggies like zucchini, carrots, asparagus, eggplant and parsnips. Spray with salt, olive oil, and paper and bake at 400 degrees up until soft.

- You could include water or veggie stock to cooked squash, potatoes or cauliflower and mash or whip. Utilize pepper and salt to taste. Miso broth works specifically great.

- Offer a good salad as a side meal, or sticks of fresh veggies.

- Pick your favorite grain, like millet, quinoa or couscous and prepare based upon the package instructions. Season with pepper and salt and serve with your main dish. You could additionally add herbs and veggies to provide it more dietary value.

- Do not forget pickled veggies-- these make a good alternative to standard side meals.

Utilize your creativity. You could additionally serve fruit as a side meal, or vegan apple sauce.

DESSERTS

Vegan Brownies

It is essential to ensure that all of these ingredients are vegan-friendly. Yes, they even have vegan chocolate!

Ingredients:

1 cup whole wheat flour

1 cup white flour

1 cup water

1 teaspoon salt

1 cup brown sugar

3/4 cup cocoa powder for baking

1 teaspoon vanilla extract

1/2 teaspoon baking powder

1/2 cup vegetable oil

Optional: 1/2 - 1 cup sliced nuts, 1/2 - 1 cup chocolate chips

Directions:

Spray a baking sheet with nonsticking cooking spray. Mix flour, brown sugar, water, and salt. (A wire whisk works ideally). Whisk in cocoa powder, vanilla extract, vegetable oil, and baking powder utilizing a wood spoon. Spread uniformly into the baking sheet and bake at 400 for around thirty minutes, up until a toothpick placed on the sides comes out clean.

THINGS TO DO WITH FRESH FRUIT

Seasonal fresh fruit produces a good dessert. You could serve it separately or attempt any of these options:

- Create a fresh fruit salad with your preferred seasonal fruits. Season the salad with citrus juice.

- Top fresh fruit with vanilla soy yogurt.

- Include fresh fruit like sliced apple to a little baking meal. Top with brown sugar, walnuts, and cinnamon and bake at 350 up until apples are soft.

- Do the same as above, but have a go at peaches, pears, blueberries or various varieties of apples too. You could additionally experiment with the spices and the nuts. This makes a great substitute for pear, blueberry, apple, or peach cobbler or crisp.

- Grill fresh pineapple pieces or bananas. Cut the banana in half crosswise and shower with cinnamon.

Simply utilize your creativity. When you take fruit and heat it somehow, it produces a gratifying and abundant dessert.

CONCLUSION of Vegan Cooking Essentials

Whether you have actually been vegan for a while or simply starting out, now you must have a more extensive understanding of what it means to be vegan. This consists of:

- Stocking your pantry

- Concealed ingredients to stay away from

- An understanding of fundamental cooking methods

- Common foods which comprise a vegan diet

- How to create well-balanced meals

- Adapting the vegan diet plan for various health issues

- Some brand-new recipes

Regardless of why you picked the vegan way of life, this book has actually been developed as a resource which is created to take you closer to attain a fully vegan and healthy way of life.

So, what now? The vegan way of life represents a dedication to improving your health. It is, likewise, a socially mindful choice for a great deal of individuals. If you wish to lower your effect on the environment further, consume local foods whenever you are able to and definitely purchase organic. Likewise, try to keep away from genetically modified foods.

Yes, the vegan way of life could definitely improve your health. It could additionally aid to encourage a better environment for many years. Simply keep in mind that just because it is vegan does not suggest it is instantly healthy. Nevertheless, it is much easier in the vegan diet plan to make healthy choices.

Gluten-Free Eating

Guide to Starting and Sticking to a Gluten-Free Lifestyle so You Can Take Your Health and Wellbeing to a Whole New Level

By Paul Dillow

Introduction to Gluten-Free Eating

You choosing to read this book is proof that the Gluten-Free movement is gradually increasing in appeal. Individuals all over the world have actually made a decision that staying clear of gluten was not simply another diet alternative, but something that is vital to their health. This is not simply another trend that is going to lose momentum before you get time to even investigate it, and it is definitely not another insane fad diet.

This shift has actually been deemed as the most sensible method for plenty of individuals to shed pounds, take charge of their health, and begin feeling like themselves once again. However, make no mistake, this diet is not for everybody. Adhering to a Gluten-Free diet is going to lead you down a road that is certainly wrought with hardship.

The issue lies in the truth that gluten is all over! Attempting to get rid of a component that is featured in such a broad range of foods is bound to be difficult. The very first hurdle is going to be discovering the self-discipline to stop eating a fair bit of the food you have actually grown to enjoy. This sounds a lot easier than it is when the 'healthier' alternative is not as yummy. The next difficulty is going to be discovering how to get adequate quantities of the nutrients you require to remain healthy without jeopardizing your decision to stay clear of gluten. And if that wasn't enough, the majority of the foods classified as "Gluten-Free" might be more pricey than their equivalents.

Whatever you choose, constantly keep in mind that your body is your home. If you do not make an effort to look after it, where are you going to live? Making an effort to eat right, exercise, and get enough rest are going to constantly be good choices. Executing effectively and at the highest level of your efficiency are going to just be possible if you look after yourself. This may need a bit more time and a little bit more effort, however, it is going to definitely be worth it.

Regrettably, there is no 'one size fits all' when it concerns our wellness and health. You need to put in the work yourself and examine your own distinct requirements. You are never ever going to have the ability to pour from an empty cup. So trust me, spend some time learning what your bodily requirements are.

By now, you ought to be questioning if all the hassle is truly worth it. And once again, I urge you to think thoroughly about whether this diet plan is actually appropriate for you. This diet plan might not be quite what you require. If it is, nevertheless, the advantages are going to far surpass any difficulties you deal with as a result of going down this path. I hate to sound sensational, however cutting gluten from your diet plan might even save your life. In order for you to be certain that this diet plan is appropriate for you, please keep on reading on to find out more about gluten and why staying clear of it is such a biggie. This might very well wind up being among the most important decisions you have actually ever made.

Chapter 1-- What is Gluten?

Simply put, gluten is among the proteins discovered in cereal grains like rye, wheat and barley. Gluten is made by a mix of 2 various proteins. These proteins are Glutenin and Gliadin. The plant depends on its supply of gluten due to the fact that it works as food for the plant throughout growth. When these grains are ground into flour, the gluten is in charge of the elasticity of dough mixes.

It is this flexibility that offers our food a particular "chewiness." People who struggle with Gluten intolerance are frequently urged to stay clear of oats too. This is since oats can quickly be tainted by foods that contain gluten, considering that it is typically processed in factories that produce food utilizing wheat and other foods that contain gluten. Some instances of gluten-free grains are sorghum, millet, buckwheat, brown rice, quinoa, wild rice, and corn.

Wheat is frequently utilized to make the following foods:

- Pasta
- Bread
- Sauces
- Baked goods
- Soups
- Cakes
- Battered meat, fish and poultry
- Salad dressings

Rye is utilized to make foods like:

- Cereals
- Pumpernickel bread
- Beer

Barley is frequently utilized to make:

- Food coloring
- Beer
- Malt milk
- Yeast
- Soups
- Malt vinegar

A lot of the foods we consume might additionally consist of some quantity of gluten as a result of being polluted throughout the manufacturing procedure. These foods consist of:

- Candy
- Dried fruit
- Caramel color
- Flavored coffee

- French fries

- Food starch

- Vegetable and meat stock

- Processed meats and cheese

- Dietary Supplements like multivitamins

- Bouillon cubes

- Ice cream

This list is not comprehensive. Time is not going to allow me to note all the foods which have or don't have gluten, and even if I had the time, you would deem it rather dull. The only effective means to figure out if your food includes gluten is to read the label thoroughly. This is going to need a great deal of your time in order for you to be precise. This comprehensive procedure might not be right for everybody.

Chapter 2—Why All the Fuss?

A current study highlighted that about 30% of all Americans are actively attempting to remove gluten from their diet plan. This are plenty of individuals when we consider the reality that there are over 330,000,000 individuals in the United States. However, why are they making such a fuss? Let's take a look at a few of the reasons why many individuals have actually chosen to live Gluten Free.

1. Celiac Disease

Research studies have actually shown that the number of people who presently struggle with this disease is on the increase. Although no official numbers have actually been released, it is approximated that well over 1% of the world's population experiences this disease. Celiac disease is specifically prevalent amongst the senior people. Even worse is the reality that lots of cases of people who struggle with this disease have actually gone undiagnosed. Actually, about

80% of individuals who struggle with celiac disease are not even cognizant that they have it.

However, exactly what is celiac disease you may be asking yourself? As emphasized in the last chapter, gluten is made up of 2 primary proteins, Glutenin and Gliadin. People with Celiac Disease react adversely to Gliadin. Celiac is categorized as an autoimmune illness. That is due to the fact that the immune system of these people tends to confuse gluten with something unsafe like a bacteria of some kind. Consequently, their bodies attempt to protect themselves from the gluten and wind up hurting themselves while doing so. This attack can lead to the degeneration of the intestinal wall and could be dangerous if not dealt with.

Other signs of Celiac Disease consist of:

- Anemia

- Nutritional shortages

- Throwing up

- Chronic fatigue

- Abdominal pain

- Abdominal bloating

- Digestive problems

- Diarrhea

- Scratchy skin rashes

- Reduced hunger

- Depression

- Irritability

- Damaged tooth enamel

- Osteoporosis

- Heartburn

- Joint pain

2. Gluten Sensitivity

Others, who do not experience Celiac Disease, have actually decided to stay clear of gluten or cut it out of their diet plan completely due to the fact that they struggle with Gluten Sensitivity. These people might have even gotten a negative result when they undertook a blood test for celiac, however, you just do not feel good when they take in foods which contain gluten. They might even struggle with signs that are rather comparable to those of somebody who has celiac disease.

Struggling With gluten sensitivity indicates that the person responds adversely to gluten despite the fact that their immune system is not harming their bodies. The signs of gluten sensitivity are normally unrelated to the intestinal tract, and they don't induce any damage to the intestinal tracts whatsoever. On the contrary, these people are more likely to experience joint pain, tiredness, abdominal pain, and even 'brain fog.' The good news is that gluten sensitivity is not deadly.

3. Gluten Intolerance

Gluten intolerance is additionally not deadly. It is going to, nevertheless, induce a fair bit of pain. People with this condition can not digest or process foods which contains gluten. This could be for a range of reasons. That person's body might not be able to produce the enzyme required to digest foods which contain gluten. Signs of gluten intolerance are generally digestion associated and might consist of bloating, gas, nausea, or diarrhea. Simply consider the outcome of eating dairy when you're lactose intolerant.

You ought to now have the understanding that living gluten-free is a really major matter for some people, and it is not a decision to be sneezed at. You are going to have the ability to value the severity of the matter, specifically if you experience these signs also. Chapter 3 of this book is about figuring out if you have any of the major gluten associated conditions that have actually been pointed out.

Chapter 3-- How to Diagnose Gluten Sensitivity, Celiac Disease and Gluten Intolerance

The significant problem with identifying whether you have gluten sensitivity, celiac disease, or gluten intolerance is that the signs look a lot like those you would have if you struggled with other illnesses. And since gluten is present in such a wide array of foods, it is simple to confuse these problems with your body merely responding adversely to a specific kind of food. That is why I would never ever urge anybody to attempt and diagnose themselves. Celiac disease can be deadly if left unattended and if the proper actions are not taken to minimize its impacts.

Although gluten intolerance and sensitivity are not deadly conditions, neglecting the signs can induce damage to your body over time. Leave the testing to the specialists. Consider how harmful it would be if you 'under-diagnosed' yourself as being gluten-sensitive when you really have celiac disease. Despite the fact that you are going to be leaving the last medical diagnosis to the specialists, it still would not hurt to find out more about the procedure.

Celiac Disease Diagnosis

A blood test is frequently utilized to validate whether your signs are due to celiac disease. Keep in mind That celiac disease happens when your body confounds the protein in gluten called Gliadin as a hazardous compound and attacks it. Your immune system is created to generate a protein referred to as an antibody so as to eradicate any organism your body thinks to be harmful. This is additionally the case when you struggle with celiac disease.

Your body is going to produce particular antibodies so as to protect itself from gluten. Blood tests are, therefore, carried out to check if your body is generating the antibodies that are specific to combating gluten. Physicians typically check for high levels of the antibody referred to as Immunoglobulin A (IgA) anti-tissue transglutaminase.

Diagnosing Gluten Intolerance or Gluten Sensitivity

Among the simplest ways for physicians to figure out if you struggle with gluten intolerance or gluten sensitivity is to ask you to do away with gluten from your diet plan for a duration of approximately 1 month. If your signs vanish or end up being less considerable during the time you stay clear of gluten, and these signs come back when you reinstitute gluten into your diet plan, then it is apparent that your body is responding adversely to gluten. A blood test can additionally be utilized to figure out if you experience either one of these conditions.

Drawbacks of the Medical System

Gluten was not a huge deal 10 years back. Physicians are even more worried about enhancing their procedure for diagnosing Cancer and STDs. Far less time is committed to investigating negative reactions to consuming gluten. Consequently, even well-meaning physicians merely confuse the signs of gluten intolerance or celiac disease with another thing.

Screening for celiac disease is most likely going to be among the last things your physician is going to suggest. In addition, there has actually been a significant quantity of cases of Physicians under diagnosing their patients' signs. Chapter 4 of this book is going to discuss how you can assist your physician to precisely diagnose you.

Chapter 4-- How to Make it Easier for Your Physician to Make a Diagnosis

As emphasized in the prior chapter, your physician is not without fault. I am not urging you to mistrust any physician who has comprehensive training and years of experience. I am, nevertheless, urging you to lend them a hand. About 14% of all medical diagnoses are false. And regardless of the very best efforts of our hard-working physicians, this is additionally true when it comes to cases which entail an adverse response to gluten. The good news is, there is a lot you can do to assist your physician in making the very best diagnosis.

Here are my recommendations:

Keep a Food Journal

By now, it ought to be rather apparent that your signs relate to your diet plan. This is often the case when your signs relate to your intestinal system. Keeping a food journal demands that you monitor the foods you consume and how frequently you consume them. In an effort to be as precise as possible, I would additionally urge you to write down the amount in which you take in these foods.

This type of information is going to provide your physician with a clear idea of the kind of food which might or might not be triggering your signs. I would urge you to do this for about 2 weeks prior to your visit. This is going to spare you a lot of time due to the fact that the majority of physicians frequently advise that you keep a precise food journal prior to making a medical diagnosis.

Write Down Your Signs

Your physician may be understanding, however, they definitely can not actually feel your pain. They are not going to have the ability to make a precise medical diagnosis if they can not isolate your signs. That is why you have to help them comprehend what you are feeling. Documenting your signs is going to be a vital gift to your physician since it is going to assist him/her in dismissing a number of unassociated conditions in a matter of minutes. Prepare a list of all your signs and the frequency of their appearance. It would additionally be great to include whether these signs happen at a particular time, like when you are doing some kind of exercise.

Be as particular as possible. For instance, please do not tell your physician that your stomach is in pain. Where does it hurt? Is it in your lower abdominal area? Is the pain acute? How long does the discomfort last? Expect the type of questions your physician is going to have to ask and write down the answers to the questions as specifically as possible. Offering this sort of information is going to spare both you and your physician a great deal of time.

In some cases, it is when we point out one particular sign or series of signs that assist the physician in piecing together the puzzle of your disease. And isn't it true that we often forget to state a few of our signs to our physicians? This is going to guarantee you say all that you have to say without needing to spend the entire day with your physician.

Inform your Physician of Other Medical Conditions

If you experience other health problems, you might have signs that might lead your physician to make an inaccurate medical diagnosis. Providing him/her with the clearest understanding of your present medical status is the very best method to assist him or her in making the very best medical diagnosis. You are going to additionally assist your physician not to squander time looking into treatments for a condition for which you have actually already gotten medication. Providing your physician with a list of your existing medications is additionally a great idea. That is going to guarantee that your physician does not recommend something that is not going to mix with your present medication.

Your physician might have to change your existing medication in order to deal with whatever brand-new condition he has actually determined. Your physician might additionally have to advise some changes to your diet plan if gluten is, in fact, impacting you adversely. He/she is going to have to have a clear image of how changing your diet plan is going to impact how your body responds to your existing medication and make the very best suggestion.

Inform your Physician of the Medical History of Your Family

Your household's medical history acts as a map to your own medical status. You are fairly likely to struggle with conditions that prevail amongst your family members. This is specifically accurate when it comes to your moms and dads who have the greatest impact on your health. Do not hesitate to ask. Our family members, specifically the males, might want to appear strong in our eyes; however, finding out about their health problems can save you.

Be on Time For Your Session

Although this is a little unrelated, I believe it has to be stated that we are frequently not too mindful of our physician's time. Appearing for a session late is going to put your physician in an extremely uncomfortable position. They are going to either need to force you to wait or infringe on the time of another individual. In either case, this is an extremely inconsiderate act and you should do your best not to place your physician in such a position. We are all really busy individuals, however, intentionally squandering the time of individuals responsible for saving lives is rather reprehensible. If you need to be late because of some inescapable disaster, I highly urge you to call the physician's office and notify them as early as possible. This is going to give them ample time to thoroughly reorganize their schedule so as to accommodate other individuals who might be waiting. The physician might even have the ability to utilize this time to take a well required and definitely, a well-deserved break.

Have Patience

Awaiting a medical diagnosis might appear to take forever. Some have actually even portrayed it as the longest wait of their lives. The minutes, hours, and even days that might go by might be painful, however, please remain patient. Bugging your physician is going to get you nowhere fast. Some things, such as the queue of blood samples waiting to be evaluated at the laboratory, are merely out of your physician's control. Enable them peace of mind and the time required to reach the most precise conclusion.

So far, we have actually explored what gluten is, how it adversely impacts some people, and even how to determine if it is damaging you. Next, we are going to turn our focus to the advantages of staying with a gluten-free diet plan.

Chapter 5-- What are the Good Things About Gluten-Free Life?

It goes without stating that eating a Gluten-Free diet plan is going to be extremely beneficial to those people who experience the gluten-associated diseases pointed out in the previous chapters. For some, this may be as easy as staying clear of stomach pain or those scratchy bumps or as significant as saving your life. Whatever the case might be, the advantages are going to speak for themselves. However, eating Gluten-free goes far beyond assisting us in staying clear of whatever signs we might have when we eat gluten. Let us take a look at these benefits from another viewpoint.

First of all, cutting gluten from your diet plan is going to push you to pay really careful attention to the foods you have actually been consuming. As soon as somebody chooses to stay clear of gluten at all costs, they are going to have to begin looking at labels and asking relevant questions.

As pointed out in chapter 1, it is simple to recognize the foods which clearly include gluten, like bread, however, how are you going to know if your dried fruits have been sprayed with a component which contains wheat in order to enhance the taste? Do you believe that grocery store attendants and restaurant owners are going to hurry to your side when they believe you will eat or buy something which contains gluten? Do you believe they want you to stop purchasing their items?

Obviously not! Your life remains in danger, so you have to step up and take all the required safety measures. When you start to inspect the labels of the foods you consume a bit more vigilantly, you are going to start to see how dreadful certain components in our foods are. Some foods include synthetic flavors, hazardous preservatives, and chemicals you would rather not take in. You are going to be stunned to see that gluten is not the only villain in your food.

These hazardous ingredients are typically carcinogenic and can result in major damage to our bodies with time. These stunning discoveries are going to drive you to look for natural options, and therein lays another advantage of the gluten-free diet plan.

The very best option for this kind of diet plan is to stay clear of excessively processed foods. A lot of pastas and bread, for instance, are created with bleached wheat and other harmful compounds. A number of the gluten-free alternatives are going to be created from other, more wholesome whole grains that have actually been processed only enough for the food to be pleasurable, however, not excessively so that they have actually protected as much of the nutrients in the food as feasible.

Extremely processed foods are additionally infamous for consisting of unhealthy oils too. Hence, a gluten-free diet plan, when given careful consideration, is going to assist you to additionally stay clear of the host of diseases connected with consuming excessive, extremely processed carbs and oils.

Numerous people who have actually chosen to stay with a gluten-free diet plan have actually found themselves consuming even more fresh vegetables and fruits than they would have taken in had they not been on this particular diet plan. A diet plan abundant in an assortment of healthy foods is constantly one that comes strongly suggested. Taking in more vegetables and fruits is going to assist in reinforcing your immune system and offering you an amazing quantity of energy to deal with every day. Taking in a diet plan this wholesome is going to additionally assist you in keeping a healthy body weight if you additionally put in the time to get routine exercise and enough rest.

Individuals who are brand-new to a specific diet plan, frequently grumble that they deal with most difficulties and temptations when they choose to eat in restaurants. Usually, the waiter is uninformed or too occupied to describe whether your meal is going to include gluten.

Furthermore, cross-contamination is a really strong possibility in these circumstances and can pose a major danger, particularly to those with celiac disease.

These problems end up being a lot more troublesome when you are eating in a group. You do not wish to seem like the weird one, and you definitely do not wish to piss off the waiter that is going to be serving your food. Due to these obstacles, numerous gluten-free zealots have actually decided to eat in restaurants less. Eating in your home regularly is going to provide these people with complete control over what they consume. You now have the choice to make tasty meals that are going to have no irritating side effects. I am not urging you to be antisocial, I am just describing what has actually worked for other folks who are in our shoes. Plus, consuming home-cooked meals is going to be good for you in many ways.

Advantages of eating at home:

- Places you in control of the portion sizes of your food

- Saves Cash

- You can feel confident that your food is prepped in a sanitary environment

- Exceptional possibilities for family bonding while the food is being prepped and eaten

There is additionally some cutting-edge research that is presently happening, which highlights that there is a connection between eating gluten-free and autism. Research studies have actually demonstrated that eating gluten-free has actually reduced the signs of autism for some kids. There is still a great deal of clashing reviews about the findings of research of this kind. It is, nevertheless, rather notable, that lots of kids' hospitals have actually reported seeing an enhancement in the social skills and behavior of kids with autism who have actually been moved to a gluten-free diet plan.

There is no question in my mind that eating gluten-free is a terrific idea if you experience any gluten-associated condition. Ideally, you too are going to be persuaded that this is an excellent idea for yourself. Please nevertheless pay close attention to the next chapter of this book due to the fact that, just like any choice, there are drawbacks when it comes to cutting gluten from your diet plan too.

Chapter 6-- Risks of Gluten-Free Eating

Among the significant problems with starting the journey of a gluten-free diet plan is that lots of people who start this journey just do not comprehend what they are entering into. They merely dive headfirst into this choice, believing it is simply another weight loss diet trend or another healthy diet plan alternative. While the advantages of this diet plan are apparent, you have to thoroughly evaluate whether this is appropriate for you. Even if you struggle with a properly diagnosed gluten-associated health problem, ample forethought ought to be given to what you do next.

2 of the risks connected with not thoroughly planning your gluten-free program that are typically highlighted are:

1. Losing out on important nutrients

2. Taking in unhealthy gluten-free foods

People who have actually chosen to take part in the gluten-free program for whatever reason without thoroughly considering their alternatives, frequently wind up losing out on essential nutrients. In spite of whatever medical conditions or goals you might have about your perfect body, health ought to constantly be our primary focus. It is inconceivable to stay healthy without a well-balanced diet plan.

A person has a well-balanced diet plan when they make an effort to take in the advised quantity of the vital nutrients our bodies require daily. Taking in an excessive or insufficient amount of any one nutrient is not going to serve to your benefit in the long run, even if you accomplish the objective of losing some excess weight.

The danger of winding up lacking in particular nutrients ends up being really genuine to those who adhere to a gluten-free diet plan due to the fact that they have actually considerably cut down on their choices. Gluten is featured in such a wide array of foods that removing it from your diet plan is going to need a lot of changes. Plenty of those who venture to stay clear of gluten are really busy individuals and have lots of clashing obligations.

This hectic world needs rather a great deal of our time, and we frequently need to sacrifice sleep simply to get all the things done. Consuming a nutritious diet plan was already really hard, and now you have actually chosen to additionally complicate your regimen by choosing to live gluten-free.

The outcome of this mix of having an excessive amount of things to do, and very few choices is going to lead to one of these 3 things. The person might wind up consuming a great deal of 'gluten-free fast foods.' They might additionally wind up just eating the identical things repeatedly. They might additionally wind up simply giving up entirely. If you started this journey since you struggle with celiac disease or another gluten-associated condition, stopping is simply not a possibility. You need to discover an approach to make this diet plan work for the benefit of your health, and in some cases, even your life.

Sadly, the other alternatives that I pointed out weren't such great ideas either. Consuming identical things repeatedly is going to suggest that you are taking in the identical nutrients constantly. This type of uniformity is going to make sticking to this diet plan extremely tough since you aren't going to delight in eating the identical thing so frequently. Consuming the identical foods constantly might not seem like such a bad thing, however, simply think of the nutrients that you are missing out on when you eat in such a manner.

In some cases, it is that one nutrient that is missing from our diet plan that makes the distinction in your health. For instance, a number of gluten-free bread alternatives frequently utilize alternatives to wheat, which include far less dietary fiber. Dietary supplements may assist in reducing the impacts of those sorts of eating practices, however, this is never ever the best choice. It is going to take some amount of preparation on your part to get the appropriate mix of nutrients.

Another significant obstacle numerous people deal with due to choosing to live gluten-free is that they end up being puzzled about the type of foods that are really beneficial to their health. Since this movement is getting momentum, sly marketing execs have actually been tagging many things as gluten-free. I have even noticed gluten-free labels on bottles of water. Sending out such a hoodwinking of a message can just serve to hurt the customers.

To make matters worse, a great deal of the foods which are being offered as Gluten-free are, in fact, really bad for your health. So as to make these foods tastier, the manufacturers frequently add a great deal of sugar or fat. A great deal of these gluten-free foods are frequently over-processed too. That is why I can not stress enough how essential it is for you to read the labels of all the things you consume. Inspect the calorie, sugar and fat content of each product. Do not make the error of presuming these products benefit your health just as long as they are tagged 'gluten-free.' As highlighted in a previous chapter, you need to watch out for your own best interest. These sly suppliers frequently do not have your best interest in mind.

This information isn't made to terrify you. However, your health is a very severe matter. If you are not cautious, your life may be at stake. You can never ever be too cautious with what you take into your body. Take the utmost precaution with anything you mean to consume, regardless of how healthy it may seem. Put in the time to do some investigation on anything brand-new or that may appear suspicious. When in doubt, adhere to natural options. You can never ever fail with ground provisions, fresh fruits and veggies. However, it could be very hard to find out how to delight in consuming healthy foods. That is why the last chapter is going to offer you a couple of easy dishes to assist you in getting going.

Chapter 7-- How to Delight In Gluten-Free Eating

Consuming a Gluten-free diet plan does not need to be dull. As formerly highlighted, staying with any diet plan is going to end up being more troublesome if you push yourself to consume identical things repeatedly. This is not going to drive you to stay with your diet plan. And the minute you see anything that resembles a challenge, you are going to quit. Sadly, quitting is not a possibility if you have gluten sensitivity, celiac disease, or gluten intolerance. Your life and your health are in question, and you have to continue going.

Here are my recommendations to keep yourself encouraged to stay with this diet plan:

1. Mix it Up!

This is the primary step to delighting in your Gluten-free journey. Do not hesitate to attempt brand-new things. If in doubt, look at the label or do some research on the web. When you are sure it does not include any gluten, dig in! Integrate it into meals you currently take pleasure in. Mixing it up is going to additionally require that you attempt brand-new recipes. Your meals ought to resemble a masterpiece. This does not indicate they need to be fancy, they just have to be enticing to the eyes. Integrate a range of various colors, textures, and flavors. Do not be upset if you fall short a couple of times prior to getting it right. This is all part of the journey.

2. Do Not Cut the Carbs!

This may appear like a rational step to feature in any diet plan. That is, nevertheless, when you are making the error of presuming that gluten-free diet plan is similar to any other diet plan.

Constantly bear in mind that your objective is merely to stay clear of foods with gluten. Carbohydrates are not the enemy. As soon as you have actually done your homework to identify if the food is safe, dig in.

3. Treat Yourself

I additionally highly suggest that you treat yourself every so often. This is another method to stay clear of making this diet plan feel difficult or uninteresting. Gluten-free treats are rather simple to discover and are just as satisfying. Now that your choices are a bit more restricted, you may additionally wish to think about different nuts and fruits as a reward. Yogurt treats and dried fruits, for instance, are simply magnificent, and there are a lot more choices to select from. You may even have choices like these as routine treats in between meals.

4. Do not Starve Yourself!

This brand-new diet plan is not going to require that you consume less calories daily. Please do not starve yourself. You may even discover yourself taking in a bit more. Some Gluten-free options, particularly those created from natural components, frequently include a lot less calories than we are used to. The outcome is that we are going to have to consume a bit more of these kinds of food in order to be pleased. Once more, there is no shame in that when you have actually performed the needed research to figure out that this food is harmless.

5. Do not be Shy!

There is no requirement to be timid about eating gluten-free. Speak out and inform your loved ones, buddies, and even the waiter serving you that you have actually picked this diet plan and describe the severity of your choice. Once they comprehend the gravity of the scenario, they too are going to end up being rather alert and assist you in keeping track of the foods you consume too. They are going to have your back and function as an additional set of eyes too.

Keep in mind, 2 heads are much better than one. And believe me, it is constantly much better to simply speak the fact than to attempt and conceal your decision or your health problem. You are going to appear quite odd when you begin staying away from the foods you once liked. Your buddies may even end up being a little concerned and presume you are on some unsafe fad diet. Calmly describing the reasoning behind it all is going to get their assistance and trust.

What you ought to take away from this chapter is that living gluten-free could be amazing and fun. Think about it as a tough brand-new food journey. You are going to be boldly moving outside your comfort zone and delving into uncharted territory. Some have actually even explained dieting as a means of feeling more in control of their lives and are thrilled to have actually established such incredible self-control.

Why should this be any different? Establishing the discipline required to cut gluten from your diet plan can offer you the self-confidence required to take charge of your life in other areas too. Whatever the case might be, delight in the trip. The following chapter is going to assist you in finding out a little bit more about the foods you can eat.

Chapter 8-- So ... What Should You Eat

Do not make the error of presuming that as soon as you change to a gluten-free diet plan, your life is over. Even if you are a food lover, you can still take pleasure in a wide array of tasty and obviously, healthy meals too. All you have to do is modify your point of view.

Rather than looking around and picturing obstacles, take a look at all the brand-new possibilities. This is a chance for you to end up being more selective and more imaginative with your food. Initially, take a cautious look at all the things that you are ablc to cat with complete confidence that they are gluten-free:

- Unprocessed Seeds (eg. chia, pumpkin and flax seeds).

- Unprocessed Beans

- Raw nuts.

- Veggies.

- A lot of dairy items.

- Eggs.

- Fish.

- Meat.

- Fruits.

- Poultry.

- Gluten-free flours (these could be created from beans, potato, soy, rice, or corn).

- Quinoa

- Hominy corn.

- Millet.

- Tapioca.

- Olive oil.

- Potatoes.

- Ghee.

- Coconut oil.

- Rice.

- Sorghum.

- Teff.

- Soy.

- Wine.

- Cider.

- Port.

- Sherry.

Alternatives to Bread:

- Brown Rice Bread.
- Millet chia bread.
- Ciabatta bread.
- Bhutanese Red Rice Bread.

Alternatives to Pasta:

- Corn Spaghetti.

- Quinoa Pasta.

- Rice-flour penne.

- Spaghetti al Riso.

Although these foods are naturally gluten-free, you still have to be careful. This is specifically so if you have actually not prepped the food yourself. You still have to take notice of just how much calories you take in and just how much fat and sugar you are consuming. Please bear in mind that not everything that is labeled gluten-free is really great for you.

Stay clear of any meat, poultry or fish that has actually been marinated, breaded, coated, or battered. You can never ever be too certain what they included in that combination. It would additionally be a great idea to avoid nuts and legumes that have been processed, and also look at the labels thoroughly prior to consuming them. You can never ever be too sure what was utilized to boost the taste.

Luckily, eating out is still a possibility. Due to all the attention the gluten-free diet plan is getting, numerous gluten-free dining establishments have actually been turning up. Do a fast Google search to determine if there are any in or near your neighborhood. You might even think about launching a business of your own too. Gluten-free dining and even gluten-free support systems are guaranteed to draw in individuals to your facility.

Your gluten-free diet plan is going to impact every part of your life. Please attempt to bear in mind that some medication is going to additionally have gluten too. If you are considering a brand-new physician, make certain to describe that you have actually cut gluten from your diet plan and the explanation for doing so. It additionally goes without stating that you are going to have to look at the labels on your nonprescription drugs really thoroughly too.

Chapter 9-- Simple Gluten-Free Options

Start yourself off with a basic 7-day meal plan. There is no requirement to figure all of it out at the same time. You have time. Consider the foods you currently delight in, determine all the possible sources of gluten, and attempt to remove them. Start simple, and after that, advance from there.

Consider this:

Monday

Meal 1: Scrambled eggs and hash browns

Meal 2: Velvety potato salad with cashews

Meal 3: Ginger and garlic aubergine steak with sweet potato wedges

Tuesday

Meal 1: Gluten-free banana pancakes with agave syrup and blended berry topping

Meal 2: Gluten-free bacon burger

Meal 3: Butter bean stew and meatballs

Wednesday

Meal 1: Breakfast smoothie with fruits of your selection

Meal 2: Sliced BLT salad

Meal 3: Gluten-free chicken pot pie

Thursday

Meal 1: Breakfast hash with sweet potatoes, eggs, and ham

Meal 2: Gluten-free quinoa burger

Meal 3: Cilantro rice and grilled salmon

Friday

Meal 1: Banana berry topping and acai bowl

Meal 2: Gluten-free fish tacos with Mexican cheese and avocado

Meal 3: Gluten-free dumplings and chicken

Saturday

Meal 1: Broccoli and potato frittata

Meal 2: Cheesy chicken chili

Meal 3: Rice noodles and garlic chicken

Sunday

Meal 1: Roasted potato wedges with caramelized onions and tuna

Meal 2: Turkey burger in buns made of zucchini

Meal 3: Shrimp burrito bowl

These dishes consist of things we make at home already. All you have to do is spend some time investigating the gluten-free replacements for the pasta and bread we are used to. Once again, the trick is to keep it enjoyable and to simply keep going.

Consuming a gluten-free diet plan actually does not need to be convoluted. The very best part is that making a meal without gluten does not constantly need to consume a great deal of your valuable time. All you have to do is plan ahead and get some of the prepping finished in advance. Veggies could be sliced up and placed in the fridge for the week. You might even schedule your day of rest for meal prepping and merely reheat your meals as the week continues. There is no requirement to interrupt your regimen. Discover what works for you and stay with it!

Conclusion of Gluten-Free Eating

My objective was to offer you the most reasonable view of the gluten-free diet plan. Ideally, you ought to have the ability to figure out if the gluten-free diet plan is appropriate for you. What I hope you have actually taken away from this book is that if you do not have a confirmed gluten-associated condition, this might not be the very best diet plan for you. If you are attempting to slim down, there are numerous other options that include minimizing your calorie intake and getting more physical activity. However, if you do choose to continue with this journey, please don't forget to be careful.

If you struggle with celiac disease, gluten sensitivity, or gluten intolerance, I hope you found these recommendations useful. Although the advantages of this diet plan are apparent, I understand that you are going to deal with lots of difficulties. However, there is no embarrassment in requesting assistance. Get your friends and family included. The assistance of your loved ones is going to provide you with the endurance you are going to require to keep going. You might even sign up with a support group. While it is great to have your family applauding you, it would be even better to look for individuals who comprehend what you are undergoing. You might get together personally or perhaps on social networks and share experiences and recipes.

Whether you have Celiac disease or not, you need to continue going. Your health is an extremely crucial matter and you must not take these health problems gently. I do not imply to frighten you, however, a few of the signs connected with these health problems can be deadly. Bear in mind that the primary step to healing is getting your signs examined by a physician.

It is constantly advised to understand simply how major your condition is. There are some circumstances where merely changing your diet plan is not going to suffice. You might additionally require other medications too. Take the suggestions in chapter 4 really seriously due to the fact that these recommendations might make the distinction in whether your physician makes the appropriate medical diagnosis or not.

To conclude, please do not ever feel embarrassed due to your medical diagnosis. Please do not be deceived by all the junk these unethical individuals have labeled as gluten-free. And lastly, please enjoy this brand-new journey regardless of what difficulties you come across.

Green Smoothie Cleanse

Learn How to Quickly and Easily Make Green Smoothies for Weight Loss, More Energy, Clear Mind and General Health

By Paul Dillow

Chapter 1: Smoothies Can Change Your Life

Envision if you could get up every morning feeling remarkable. Rather than getting up with a headache, or having a hard time opening your eyes due to the fact that you're still so tired; you simply jump out of bed full of life and all set to go and handle the day. This energy is then enough to carry you through job and workouts. You have enough to work on tasks, to keep your home tidy and clean, and to make the most of each hour. And envision if you had the dream body you have actually constantly desired: ripped muscle, flat abs, and skin that looks radiant and healthy.

Naturally, there's no quick fix that is able to make all of this a reality, however, it is a great goal to have. And really, there are simply a couple of basic things you may do that are going to instantly take you a lot nearer to that reality. Among them is simply beginning to drink a smoothie daily.

Really? A smoothie? A drink that can enhance your health, your state of mind, your looks and your energy levels? Certainly-- and a lot more too! In this book, you'll find out how smoothies can transform your life and you'll find simple recipes for smoothies that fight stress, improve immunity, build muscle, enhance athletic functionality, battle cancer, and A LOT MORE.

Why We Require Nutrients

A smoothie is naturally a mix of various vegetables and fruits. You just take a number of fruits, drop them into a blender, and hit 'go' to ensure that your drink is going to be prepared to take in. It's a basic procedure; however, it's enough to offer you a drink that not just tastes fantastic; however, additionally offers you lots of nutrition. And this is the keyword: nutrition.

What is exceptionally crucial for everyone, is that we consume a nutrient-dense eating plan. That is to state that it isn't sufficient that we see our eating plan just as a source of fuel-- it additionally needs to provide basic materials that supply us with improved health and functionality. The old stating that you 'are what you consume' is actually correct. Your muscles, your hormones, your bones, your brain cells, your body immune system, and your digestion enzymes are all created from nutrients in your food, and that's what makes it so essential.

When you take in fruits, vegetables or meats, your body is going to continue to break them down, and after that, utilize the constituent parts to carry out many tasks throughout your system. These assist you to grow, to combat health problems and to work optimally. And it's no coincidence that we require veggies, fruits and other components to grow. Besides, these are the important things we evolved consuming. It's not that our biology required us to look for these foods-- the foods were readily available and so our biology adjusted to endure on them.

We require these ingredients to prosper and without them, we begin to actually break down. We begin to see indications of bad health like trouble sleeping, fragile hair and nails, absence of muscle tone and weaker bones. Our hormones fall out of whack and we ultimately begin to see severe diseases and other conditions gradually develop. And this isn't the exception. This isn't an uncommon and regrettable situation that just some individuals experience ... this is the standard.

A substantial amount of the illnesses and diseases that impact us in old age are really extremely preventable degenerative illness? Your body was constructed to last you your whole life. In theory, you ought to have the ability to remain healthy, engaged and active right up till you keel over. However, poor nutrition enables all sorts of issues to gradually sneak up on us from weak bones, to cardiovascular disease, to hypertension, to arthritis, to dementia. Not all of these conditions are preventable; however, in a lot of cases, they are. So what's the issue with our contemporary eating plan?

Issue With Contemporary Diets

The greatest problem is that we consume excessive refined food. What is refined food? Basically, it's food that has actually been prepared and made in such a way that it bears little similarity to the initial components. A fine example may be a sausage rolls. Here, you believe that you are obtaining some pastry and meat. The pastry is created from egg and flour, however, at least the sausage is genuine meat, loaded with actual minerals and amino acids, right? Incorrect! That meat is probably a mix of all the cast-offs from many other meals that have actually been combined together and mushed into a pulp.

That implies you're obtaining the gristle and the parts of the meat that nobody would consume in any other form. From there, the sausage meat then has massive quantities of sugar, fat and salt included. This assists to protect the sausage and ensure it still has that appealing grey color when you come to consume it.

What about the vegetables and fruits you get in your cereal and your breakfast bars? Nope, they're just as bad! These fruits have actually been 'freeze-dried.' That indicates that they have actually gone through a vacuum and sub-zero temperature levels. The low-temperature level is going to have frozen the wetness to the point that it ends up being small icicles, and the low pressure is going to remove them from the fruit by force.

You believe that will not bring with it a few of the critical nutrients along the way? Apart from anything else, when you take in something consisting of vitamin C, you require wetness so as to absorb it. Vitamin C is actually a water-soluble vitamin and you can't utilize it if it's not presented properly. And once again, a great deal of sugar and other ingredients are going to be included, which are going to make your fruit appear vibrant and edible. Something like chocolate bars or crisps, on the other hand, hardly have any nutrients in them to start with!

Why Empty Calories Are Bad

All this implies that you are taking in empty calories. An empty calorie is a food such as sausage rolls, unhealthy breakfast cereals, and all-set meals which contain a great deal of calories, yet little genuine nutrition. You're briefly filling yourself up and increasing your blood glucose; however, you're not supplying any real nourishment. Plus, these empty calories take the shape of simple carbohydrates.

Since there's absolutely nothing 'genuine' left in them, you'll absorb them too rapidly, leading to a spike in blood glucose. This offers a brief energy burst, however, that then goes just as rapidly, leaving you yearning actual food. Additionally, you'll be malnourished. And what's more, is that this is going to ultimately equate to the accumulation of more major conditions and illness.

Stopping working to get the correct food in your diet plan is additionally what triggers weight gain and snacking habits. This is partially because of the truth that your blood glucose troughs not long after it surges and partially due to the truth that your body is going to 'long for' the things it requires. If you're not getting sufficient vitamin C, then your body is going to inform you it desires something sweet. It's attempting to convey that you require an orange or an apple-- however, years of training mean that you'll translate this as wanting a chocolate bar! And even before that takes place, you'll discover you put on weight quickly, and you need to drag yourself through the day as some type of zombie! When you see food only as fuel and forget that it is likewise nourishment, that is when your body begins to fail you.

Why Smoothies Are So Good

So why are smoothies the solution? Vegetables and fruits are especially high in a lot of the micronutrients that we actually require. They additionally supply them in a way that is extremely practical, which is simple for the body to take in. And hence, when we consume smoothies, we supply a 'hit' of terrific things that are going to assist to power us through the day.

There are alternative choices, obviously. One is simply to attempt and get more home-prepared vegetables and fruits in your eating plan. This is going to certainly assist to provide all the same nutrients, however, let's be sincere-- it's likewise a great deal of effort and something a lot of us are going to fall short at.

Be sincere with yourself. Are going to you actually dedicate to cooking supper from the ground up every night? Are you truly going to adhere to your 5 fruit a day rule too? Keep in mind that the rule of 5 is arbitrary. The truth is that we require more nutrients than 5 vegetables and fruits are going to truly provide us with. It's likewise essential to keep in mind that it's more about what we're consuming than just how much.

Consuming kiwi fruits, avocados, mangos, bananas and blueberries is going to have a far different effect than consuming 5 apples-- or any other assortment of vegetables and fruits. And do not even get me begun on sauces and all set meals which do not provide any of the fiber that you'd receive from genuine fruit.

Smoothies provide a practical method to make certain you're getting a BIG helping of minerals and vitamins that are ready to go and that makes them an exceptional option that can fight a lot of the ill-effects of a contemporary eating plan. Smoothies likewise let you get a lot more imaginative and not spend hours chopping up or peeling your fruits. The other alternative option that might currently have actually crossed your mind, is to supplement so as to get your requirement of minerals and vitamins.

While this is a great alternative, it is essential to acknowledge that supplementing is never ever as reliable as obtaining the identical nutrients and minerals naturally. Once again, this boils down to our evolution and the manner in which our bodies are created to obtain nourishment. Some vitamins, for instance, are best taken in with fats, whereas others are much better taken in with water. Some get soaked up immediately, whereas others take longer to absorb.

Some minerals and vitamins work best when taken simultaneously. All these are things that numerous supplements do not take totally into account and the outcome is that a great deal of the good winds up getting flushed down the toilet. With vegetables and fruits, however, the vitamins and minerals are easily offered in a 'bioavailable form' that the body is far better at utilizing.

What To Anticipate When You Start With Smoothies

So what should you anticipate when you begin consuming smoothies frequently? As I wrote at the beginning of this chapter, you ought to anticipate to see your energy change in a BIG way. All the most energetic individuals-- all individuals who are most focussed and driven when it concerns pursuing goals and getting what they desire-- are individuals who have routine smoothies.

You can likewise anticipate to feel much better. You'll discover that your skin, nails and hair look much better, you'll discover that your eyes are whiter and individuals are going to comment that you have a 'healthy radiance.' You'll feel much healthier too. You'll sleep much better, you'll discover that you get ill much less typically and you'll discover that you have to get snacks less throughout the day. You'll slim down too, thanks partially due to the lesser consumption of food (a great side effect of decreased hunger and cravings) and partially to the boosted metabolic rate of your body that is going to assist you to burn through fat.

Most importantly, you'll be enhancing your body and enhancing your long-lasting health to ensure that you are less probable to establish cancer, Alzheimer's, cardiovascular disease or many other conditions. And this should not come as a surprise. This is no exotic supplement that is turbocharging your body. This is how you are supposed to feel. This is how we felt constantly.

Chapter 2: The Downsides and Dangers of Smoothies

Before we dive right in, however, you have to be conscious that there are some dangers and disadvantages included with smoothies too. Smoothies may do a world of good, and throughout the remainder of this book you are going to be finding out the components, the tricks and techniques to taking pleasure in some seriously delicious and healthy juices. However, regrettably, similar to any health trend, there are likewise those on the internet who are spreading incorrect info and typically inducing harm to the good name of smoothies!

The initial thing to be familiar with is the concept of 'juice fasting.' Here, individuals are going to utilize smoothies as meal substitutes and are going to just endure on juice for a duration of days or weeks. The claim is that this is an excellent method to 'detox' the body and to get rid of 'contaminants' and other things, in addition to being an excellent way to jump-start your weight loss.

This is not a great idea. As far as detoxing goes, what is essential to remember is that this is another approximate term that does not actually have any meaning. There is no scientific evidence that we have to detox by any means or that we have an 'accumulation' of contaminants.

The fact is that our body has its own system of cleansing and this works simply great without our assistance. Your body is going to have no problem in getting rid of toxic substances in time, and they are not most likely to develop or boost in number by any means. In one research study, scientists asked the makers of 'detoxing hair items' to name a few of the toxic substances that their hair shampoos might fight-- they discovered that the makers could provide no good description.

We like the idea of detoxing due to the fact that it appears to make sense, however, the truth is that this is, in fact, simply a wild-goose chase. And what you likewise have to be familiar with is the high sugar material discovered in smoothies. Now, sugar is not constantly a bad thing and throughout this book, you are going to find out to alleviate the sugar discovered in your smoothies. Nevertheless, when you get rid of the food from your diet plan, you get rid of the buffer to shield you from the acidity and sugars of your smoothies.

This can then lead to some major damage to health and an eating plan consisting simply of smoothies is most likely to harm the stomach lining,and more significantly: the teeth. I, in fact, know somebody who attempted a 'smoothie fast' and they wound up wearing away all of the enamel from their teeth. They needed to go to the physician and lost 2 teeth after simply one week. So think hard and long prior to getting on board any juice fasts or other fads.

The last thing to think of is whether an eating plan is maintainable. If you are going to 'begin' an eating plan by utilizing an extraordinary fast, then you'll be placing your body through hell just to go back to a typical kind of eating. That suggests your weight is going to merely go back to what it was prior to the fast and you will not have benefited.

Additionally, when you fast for this long, you really boost your possibility of keeping fat. Many procedures in the body guarantee this, however, one crucial example is that your body is going to generate a great deal of cortisol to respond to low blood glucose. This cortisol then promotes lipogenesis-- the development of brand-new fat deposits. Oh, and it likewise ruins muscle, and that makes you less metabolically active. It diminishes testosterone considerably too, which additionally decreases your metabolic process.

However, you're getting sugar right? From all that fruit? Yes - however, just simple sugar. Fruits soak up extremely rapidly into the bloodstream which implies that you're going to be obtaining 3 enormous spikes of energy across the day and absolutely nothing more. This is bad for your insulin level of sensitivity and it implies you are extremely likely to keep all that sugar as fat. So simply put: stay away from smoothie 'cleanses' and juice fads. Rather, concentrate on including smoothies into your eating plan!

How to Prevent Harming Yourself With the Sugar in Smoothies

Smoothies do a lot of good, however, as we have actually found out, they can additionally bring a couple of dangers with them. If you're now worried about the prospective damage that the sugar in smoothies may do, it may have put you off of the concept of including smoothies to your eating plan. However, do not stress-- when you include simply one smoothie of an affordable size to your morning regimen, you have absolutely nothing to fret about.

This is true if you additionally ensure that you minimize sugar from other sources in your diet plan. If you have especially delicate teeth though, or if you do not respond well to sugar, another choice is to concentrate more on veggie smoothies or to search for fruits that are lower in sugar. There are a lot of great choices to pick from and including more water to your smoothie can additionally assist to dilute it. When we go through the recipes and ideas, you'll see that there are a variety of various choices that are lower in sugar than average.

Chapter 3: Making the Perfect Smoothie

First, we're going to take a look at the fundamentals that apply to any smoothie. Due to the fact that truly, you do not always require a recipe. There's absolutely nothing incorrect with simply trying out various mixes of vegetables and fruits and tweaking the ratios to discover things you like.

Somewhere else in this book, you'll discover a guide to the various health advantages of numerous vegetables and fruits, in addition to the advantages of various nutrients-- that can act as an excellent beginning point. However, to get imaginative, you have to understand the fundamental guidelines. How do you ensure that your smoothie is 'essentially delicious' and does not leave you cold?

The Essentials

The initial thing to do is to pick the vegetables and fruits that you're going to include in your smoothie. As pointed out, you ought to select the vegetables and fruits based upon the objectives you wish to attain and the nutrients that you have an interest in. Obviously, you ought to go for a balance.

Think about the acidity and sugar content. Something like avocado or banana is going to be much less sweet than something like mango or orange. If you have a couple of components that pack a great deal of sugar, then think about including a couple of less sweet components to attempt and even the score. What's additionally extremely crucial, is to make certain that you hit your ratios.

Liquid

The first thing to include prior to making your smoothie is some type of liquid. What's additionally crucial, though, is that you consider just how much liquid you desire and what kind of liquid you're going to utilize. The most typical option of liquid is going to be water. Nevertheless, it's additionally relatively typical to utilize milk (which comes loaded with its own nutrients) or to utilize fruit juices. It's additionally typical to utilize 1 to 2 cups for someone's worth of smoothie.

Keep in mind, though, that your smoothie's consistency is quite dependant on what you do now. If you desire the drink to be extremely runny, then including a great deal of water and juice is great. If you choose a thicker consistency, however, then you'll wish to include a little less and/or pick something that is more thick to start with like milk or perhaps yogurt. Whether you choose your drink to be runny or thick is your decision and may additionally differ depending upon the goal and the recipe! Typical liquids you can utilize for tasty smoothies consist of:

- Water

- Almond milk

- Milk

- Coconut milk

- Coconut water

- Organic fruit juice

- Newly squeezed juice

- Kefir

- Tea

- Yogurt

Have a good time and experiment!

Base

The following thing to consider is your base texture. This is what will offer the body of your smoothie and provide it that solid consistency to ensure that it is a smoothie and not a juice. The goal here is to select something that has a more thick consistency itself then and that implies something along the lines of mangos, bananas, peaches, peaches or avocados. Yogurt likewise works effectively, as do nut butters (such as peanut butter), chia seeds, coconut oils, ice, frozen fruit and even ice cream (though this last possibility is not so healthy!).

Excellent bases consist of:

- Mangos

- Bananas

- Peanut butter

- Pears

- Yogurt

- Avocado

- Peaches

- Frozen fruit

- Apples

- Melon

- Plums

The Ratios

The following thing to do is to place the extra fruits and/or veggies in the needed ratios. You have actually currently set them aside, now you have to select the particular amounts and include them in. For example, if you're going to create a green smoothie, then you'll most likely be including kale, spinach, beet greens, lettuce, dandelions, cauliflower, broccoli, and so on. For juicy ones, you'll probably have things such as oranges, berries, apples, and so on.

You currently have your base, and this will offer the most flavor to start with. Selecting fruits from here then is a matter of selecting what matches that base, and you can work this out by considering what works good on a plate together!

For instance, a terrific dessert is to have berries with yogurt and because of that, you can get the identical tasty result by including berries to a yogurt base. This is going to offer you lots of anti-oxidants, while the yogurt particularly will assist you in getting gastrointestinal advantages (we'll talk more about this in a subsequent chapter). On the other hand, strawberries are understood to go effectively with banana. Similarly, orange and mango is an excellent mix!

Start Mixing!

With all that done, include your fruits into the blender (de-seeded and stones), and after that, mix them up into a pulp. You can constantly include more water at this point in case you determine it requires it. Keep in mind to keep your hand over the cover!

How to Obtain More From Your Smoothies

These directions are going to assist you to begin trying out your own smoothies and feeling the health advantages of obtaining more minerals and vitamins for yourself. However, there are likewise a variety of other things you may do to create your meals that much more delicious, to make them more enjoyable or to spare time. Here are some pointers:

Include Garnishes

There are various garnishes you can include in a smoothie if you wish to provide a more excellent taste and appearance. For instance, you can spray some sliced nuts or granula on the top and this is going to assist to fill you up. Nuts are additionally a terrific option if you are going to be utilizing peanut butter as a base!

Sweeteners

If you think that your smoothie isn't sweet enough, then you may be lured to include some sugar or a syrup/sweetener. This isn't an especially excellent idea. Sugarcoating your smoothie is naturally just going to intensify the problems currently connected with the high sugar material in these beverages. On the other hand, sweeteners, in fact, 'deceive' the body into believing it has actually taken in sugar and set off an insulin reaction-- which in turn triggers us to feel exhausted and might be bad for our health.

There are some alternatives that individuals choose (like stevia); however, on the whole, it's much better to stick to natural components: simply include more of the sweeter fruits and possibly think about utilizing some honey. Honey, in fact, has a lots of advantages and is terrific prior to bed!

Chapter 4: Fitting Smoothies Into Your Regimen

What's, in fact, equally as essential as discovering to make smoothies, is finding out how to fit them into your regimen. Previously, we talked about how you might repair your eating plan simply by intending to get more vegetables and fruits in it naturally. Obviously, this is an easy option and is equally as healthy as having vegetables and fruits.

The issue, as we saw, was that a great deal of individuals have a hard time fitting that into their regimen. They start with excellent objectives; however, it just takes a long day at work for preparing a meal to be off the table (pun intended). Similarly, if you're on the train and all you can purchase for lunch is a refined sandwich, that will not leave you with much options except to break the healthy eating plan.

Smoothies work since they're simpler to fit into a typical regimen. However, they are not completely easy, and every now and then, you'll discover that they can still appear like excessive work, excessive effort and excessive mess. This is especially correct, given that you do not simply need to make the smoothie. You likewise have to clean up the smoothie maker, source the vegetables and fruits and usually put a great deal of time and work into preparing them-- and they're costly!

Our goal here then, is to make certain we are prepared up to win. You have to ensure that it is simpler to stick to your smoothie strategy than it is to cheat on it and skip them. This chapter is going to assist you to do precisely that!

What You Need

The initial thing to do is to decrease the quantity of work you have for yourself by utilizing the appropriate tools. Front and center is that smoothie maker itself! An excellent smoothie maker/blender/food processor/juicer ought to be something that is extremely effective. You wish to have the confidence of understanding that you can toss any mix of vegetables and fruits in there (reasonably) and that it will not get stuck in the procedure.

You desire it to be quick and without a mess. What's additionally extremely essential is that you decrease the quantity of washing up you need to do for yourself. The huge issue here is that healthy smoothie makers are frequently really bothersome to clean and wash. This holds true particularly thanks to their blades, that are uncomfortable to reach and which turn when you attempt and grip them.

These elements mix to make cleaning out your mixers a royal headache. Luckily, some more recent designs have actually been developed with this in mind and feature blades that are simple to take out or that do not enter direct contact with the pulp and therefore remain cleaner.

Another convenient function is the capability to eliminate the top of your mixer and go. The initial item to get well-known for doing this was the NutriBullet, however, its appeal has actually generated numerous copycats. The concept is that you have a water bottle and a blender integrated into a single item, indicating that you do not have a detached glass to wash up!

Preparation and Pick-Up

Preparation and Pick-Up is an idea that originates from author Tim Ferriss. The concept is that you wish to perform all of your work in advance, to ensure that all you need to do when it pertains to the crunch is pick it up and go. In our case, that indicates that you're going to put together your smoothie at the beginning of the week and after that consume it throughout the week. One method to do this is simply to make substantial amounts of your smoothies on a Sunday, and after that, to keep them in bottles in the refrigerator. Each early morning, you can just get a bottle and go, without needing to, in fact, work over it!

Some individuals additionally discover it practical to freeze the fruits themselves previously. This is an excellent option due to the fact that it enables them to purchase wholesale upfront, and after that, they do not stress over ripening. Bear in mind though, that ripe fruit is less of a concern when it's being mixed anyhow! You can additionally make your life a little simpler by purchasing your vegetables and fruits online. This is a terrific option if you discover you are having a hard time to get time to go out and get what you need as it suggests they are going to all be prepared for you and you can merely drop them in the mixer prepared to go.

You can additionally make savings in this manner! Keep in mind: If you have an interest in cost savings on your vegetables and fruits, then the best method to purchase is from a market. If you happen to have one close to you, then make certain you make the most of that!

Easy Smoothies

You can additionally create your smoothies a bit easier in various other methods. Utilizing a pure fruit juice, for example, can conserve time and effort, along with utilizing canned fruits and purees. These are specifically helpful for things such as pineapples, cranberries and peaches. Why? Due to the fact that those components are especially hard to prepare and include a great deal of de-seeding and peeling. By utilizing a tinned fruit, you have it prepared to go in a shape that is simple and soft to mix!

Bought Smoothie

If you actually do not have time to create your own smoothies, then should you be lured by store-bought smoothies? Is this an excellent way to get your components without investing time? The response is yes and no ... Obviously, creating your own smoothie provides you tighter control over the nutrition, it conserves you a great deal of cash, and all in all, it is a smarter option. While purchasing a store-bought smoothie may not seem like a great deal of cash (maybe setting you back $3 a day) it is going to rapidly build up, and that is, in fact, $21 a week! However, if you generally get a coffee every early morning, then you can switch it for a smoothie and shell out just as much while obtaining health advantages rather than feeding yourself with that wired sensation that you receive from coffee!

If purchasing smoothies in town is the only method by which you can persevere, then it's cash well-spent. However, do be really mindful to inspect the ingredients completely. Even if the components extol how many fresh fruits they put in, that does not imply that they have not additionally flooded it with additives, sugars and other things.

Chapter 5: Energy and Defence Smoothies

Okay, so you understand why smoothies are so great for you, you understand how to create them and you understand how to prevent the typical mistakes ... So I think it's time that we began taking a look at some actual recipes to assist strengthen your health and change your looks and energy. We're going to begin with an 'energy and defence' technique. The smoothies we're taking a look at in this chapter are everything about supplying you with great deals of energy and simultaneously, enhancing your immune system to offer you with much better defense versus disease and illness.

This is your standard smoothie and it's what many people connect with smoothies. So what should you take into a smoothie developed for energy and defence? Here is one tip:

Morning Wakeup Smoothie

To begin with, here is the recipe:

- 1 Beet

- half a cup of cold water

- 1 tablespoon honey

- Lemon juice

- 2 cups of blended frozen berries

- 2 tablespoons of coconut oil

If you're accustomed to having coffee first thing in the early morning, then you may discover that you depend on utilizing a specific thing as a pick-me-up. The issue, though, is that coffee does not have all that much dietary worth and it is addicting. Caffeine works by obstructing the receptors in the brain that react to adenosine-- which is a repressive neurotransmitter that we generate as a result of the energy procedure.

The more time we spend working, the more adenosine develops and the slower and less cognitively able we end up being. By obstructing these receptors, caffeine can stop adenosine from having any effect, and this consequently indicates that the brain feels more awake. The issue is that the brain reacts to this. How? By producing more adenosine receptors! The outcome is that you now require much more caffeine to feel its impacts.

Worse is that when you aren't taking in any caffeine, you are going to feel lethargic, slow and susceptible to headaches! When you are asleep, you naturally aren't obtaining any caffeine and some individuals now think that the early morning grogginess all of us experience (sleep inertia) is, in fact, frequently brought on by caffeine withdrawal!

Then there's the reality that caffeine promotes the release of stress hormones such as norepinephrine and cortisol. It would be a relatively precise description to state that caffeine resembles 'stress in a cup.' As you can most likely figure out by now then, coffee isn't a healthy option for an early morning increase! This smoothie, however, is, and it has lots of various components that do a world of good to wake you up in the early morning, offer you energy throughout the day and shield you from damage.

Let's analyze each component:

Berries

A mix of berries is a great method to enhance your immunity and to shield yourself versus a variety of illnesses-- cancer particularly. That's due to the fact that berries are definitely loaded with anti-oxidants. Anti-oxidants are compounds that fight the action of 'free radicals' in the body. Free radicals, on the other hand, are substances that damage cells when they enter into contact with them. These can trigger noticeable indications of aging as the damage ends up being visible in our hair and skin.

However more worrying is what occurs when those free radicals pierce our cell walls and all the way to our nuclei-- the centers of the cells which contain our DNA. When this occurs, they can harm those strands of DNA sufficiently to trigger little anomalies.

And if those anomalies are copied, this is how we get malignant growths. In other words, an eating plan high in anti-oxidants is among the greatest things you can try to find to enhance your health. Including berries in a smoothie is among the most effective methods to achieve this without a doubt.

Beet Juice

What you're actually going to feel when you consume this smoothie, however, is the power of the beet juice. Beet juice is, in fact, such a powerful efficiency enhancer that it is utilized by a variety of various professional athletes? That's due to the fact that beet juice functions as a 'vasodilator'.

A vasodilator is something that expands the capillary (arteries and veins) and thus assists more oxygen and blood to circumnavigate the body. This implies more oxygen and blood to your brain, which consequently equates to much better concentration, psychological energy and cognitive efficiency. It additionally indicates you're most likely to delight in much better energy generally and you might experience substantial functionality enhancements if you head out for a lengthy run!

Honey

Honey is a terrific option for energy due to the fact that it offers its sugar in a variety of various methods. Particularly, honey consists of both sucrose and fructose which are soaked up into the bloodstream at various rates. This implies that honey can provide you a little sugar hit right at the beginning of the day; however, it will likewise act as a slower supply to keep you going up until lunch. This can assist to avoid snacking. Obviously, honey likewise provides our smoothie a little bit of sweet taste!

Coconut Oil

Coconut oil is another extremely effective addition in this smoothie-- everything is there for a reason! Coconut oil is an excellent option due to the fact that it consists of an extremely particular kind of fat: medium-chain triglycerides. This fat is soaked up in a different way from other kinds of fat in the body and it is going to head directly to your liver, where it is going to promote the generation of ketones.

Ketones are interesting to us since they function as a 'secondary' form of energy for the body. When the body does not have glucose, it counts on ketones rather. Hence, your body can make it through on ketones, and really the brain favors ketones for particular jobs. Any mix with coconut oil is going to offer you a huge increase and is going to assist you to feel more alive and alert!

Lemon

Lastly, we have lemon juice, which is a terrific source of many minerals and vitamins, along with numerous other things. In this specific smoothie, the function of the lemon juice is to offer vitamin B6 and C, in addition to offering us that revitalizing wakeup call that you can just receive from citrus!

Stress Buster Smoothie

Not a fan of that previous smoothie? The upcoming one is going to assist to support your immunity and battle stress, however, without quite a lot of fuel for vasodilation or ketones. Once again, let's deal with the components initially:

- 1 cup organ juice

- 2 bananas

- 3/4 cup of almond milk

- 1 peeled orange

- 1 tsp vanilla extract

- Ice

- 1 carrot peeled

This is another terrific one for combating early morning tiredness and offering you some get-up and go. The bananas are a terrific source of potassium and energy, which are going to assist in sustaining you for a lot longer!

The carrot is crucial due to the fact that it consists of excellent amounts of B6 (as does the banana) and this assists the body to handle energy from food. This implies that you'll obtain more usage out of the carbohydrates that you take in and out of the very sugar in this smoothie!

Even better, recent research study recommends that lutein (which is discovered in carrots) may be helpful at enhancing the energy performance of our mitochondria. Mitochondria are the little 'energy factories' in our cells that have the job of transforming glucose and other types of energy into ATP, then utilizing that ATP to drive the motion of muscles and sustain our cells. In one research study, it was discovered that when mice were provided lutein, they would run additionally on their wheel and, in fact, burn a lot more calories-- without any prompt from the scientists! Lutein needs a source of fat since it is fat-soluble.

The bright side is that the almond milk in this smoothie is going to do that task simply perfectly. Vanilla extract, on the other hand, is another powerful anti-oxidant. In addition to offering anti-inflammatory qualities and combating cholesterol, it's a great tool for making our smoothie a bit sweeter.

Lastly, we have the orange which is actually the 'stress-busting' part of the formula. There's a great deal of orange in here and that's going to supply a great deal of vitamin C. Vitamin C plays an essential function due to the fact that it is what the brain utilizes to create serotonin. Serotonin, on the other hand, is the 'joy hormone' and our extremely own 'natural' anti-anxiety medication. By keeping your blood glucose stable and supplying serotonin, this drink can set you up in an excellent state of mind and offer the ideal start to the day!

Brain Fuel Smoothie

Got a tough day up ahead? This 'brain fuel' smoothie ought to offer your grey matter with everything it requires to ace any difficulty!

- Protein powder

- 1-2 tsp coconut oil

- 1t cinnamon

- 1/2 banana

- 1-2tsp yerba mate green tea

This mix is an effective smoothie for anybody aiming to enhance their focus and concentration. The initial thing of interest in here is the protein powder. Protein is brain food since it is where we obtain our amino acids--with amino acids being chiefs in the production of various neurotransmitters. In other words, our brain requires protein to operate correctly and protein powder is an excellent source.

Next up, we have coconut oil and banana, which we have actually currently seen the advantages of. Coconut oil particularly is important for brainpower, and it's really the essential component in a great deal of items developed to boost brain efficiency. Cinnamon, on the other hand, is an extremely healthy method to include more taste to our beverage. It reduces blood glucose and it additionally assists in lowering the possibility of heart problem. As a matter of fact, the capability of cinnamon to decrease blood glucose is so powerful, that it is typically suggested for diabetic clients. This makes it ideal for us to, once again, prevent those spikes and drops in blood glucose that can destroy our effectiveness otherwise.

Cinnamon additionally packs a great deal of anti-oxidants to assist to support the brain for the longer term. The last component here is the yerba mate green tea. Green tea is a wonderful choice for anybody wanting to improve their mental capacity and is a much better option than coffee. For starters, the caffeine material is substantially lower in green tea, which implies you can get the minor increase without fretting as much about jitters, stress and dependency. Furthermore, green tea consists of the perfect mix of l-theanine and caffeine. L-theanine has an effect on the brain that is rather the 'opposite' of caffeine because it is delicately inhibitory.

Many individuals discover that when they integrate caffeine with l-theanine, the two complement one another completely. The caffeine assists to wake individuals up and make them more focussed and alert, while the theanine assists keep them calm and stops stress levels from reaching an all-time high!

Green tea is additionally really high in anti-oxidants too. Any green tea is going to get the job done. As a matter of fact, Darwin himself is reported to have actually portrayed green tea as the ideal stimulant. It ought to additionally serve to be neuroprotective and minimize the possibility of dementia, Alzheimer's or other kinds of cognitive decrease.

Breakfast Smoothie

Lastly, let's have a look at a breakfast smoothie that has one task-- to fill you up and keep you going up until lunch for those special days!

- 150g strawberry

- 1/2 avocado

- 200ml semi-skimmed milk

- 4 tablespoon low-fat natural yogurt

- Lemon or lime

- Honey

This is a smoothie created to see you through the day up until lunch, which is going to assist improve your functionality and stop cravings. The very best part of this smoothie is the avocado, which provides a scrumptious base and which, likewise, assists to give energy really gradually throughout the day because of its status as a healthy saturated fat.

It was once believed that saturated fats would trigger heart issues and weight gain. Recently however, research studies have actually revealed that this is not the case. While saturated fats do consist of more calories, they are additionally, in fact, much better for us thanks to their sluggish release of energy, and that makes them really reliable in supplying us with a consistent supply of energy and preventing sugar spikes in the blood.

We have actually likewise seen that honey has a comparable result when it concerns discharging energy gradually. And that low-fat yogurt can assist in getting your gut germs in check, which is really essential for digestive function. This is something we are going to taking a look at in more detail in the next chapters.

Ideally, this has actually offered you a couple of ideas for fantastic early morning smoothies you can utilize to begin your day right. And by sharing the thinking behind every one and the reason they are so powerful, you are going to ideally now have a much better concept of how to get comparable results while still exploring the components as you please!

More significantly, I hope that this chapter has actually now opened your eyes to the genuine power of smoothies. We're talking game-changing enhancements in health and functionality here. These smoothies do not simply offer you a little bit of energy and nutrition-- when you stick to them, they'll assist to shield your brain as it ages, shield your cells from cancer and more. And we're simply getting going!

Chapter 6: Smoothies for Sleep, Digestion and Hangover

You have actually seen a lot of smoothies that you can count on as your early morning pick-me-up, and any of these are going to assist you to enhance your basic health while likewise assisting you to feel a lot more energetic throughout the whole day. Keep in mind: one smoothie is going to make you feel much better for a couple of hours. However, it's by consuming smoothies routinely that you begin to see the advantages develop gradually and truly alter your life. Stay with it!

That stated, you may discover you wish to explore some various components to see if you can take pleasure in a few of the many other possible advantages of smoothies. This chapter then is going to take a look at some more basic favorable health results of drinking smoothies. Particularly, we'll find how you can increase your sleep, help your food digestion and even fight a hangover!

The Bed Time Smoothie

This bedtime smoothie is going to assist you to sleep more deeply and it is going to likewise assist you to be more anabolic through the night to ensure that you put on more muscle!

- 1/2 a banana

- 2 cups whole milk

- 2 tablespoons peanut butter

- Kiwi

- Cherries

- 1 tablespoon honey

There's a lot of excellent stuff in this smoothie that is going to assist you to sleep more deeply and get up feeling more stimulated. For athletes and bodybuilders, this smoothie is going to likewise assist in placing you in a more anabolic state, indicating that you'll generate more testosterone through the night and get up with improved energy. So how does it all work?

First off the whole milk. Whole milk is a perfect option for drinking prior to bed and particularly for males. That's due to the fact that whole milk can considerably enhance testosterone generation, and most of our testosterone production takes place during sleep. Particularly, we produce the most testosterone at 4 am! Why is whole milk so essential for testosterone?

Simple: testosterone is created from healthy saturated fats. And whole milk consists of great deals of saturated fat. Ladies, on the other hand, can simply delight in the calming advantages of milk, which ought to assist to put them in the state of mind for sleep! The peanut butter remains in here partially due to the fact that it is going to offer a source of protein while you're sleeping, so your body can put that testosterone to the excellent usage and develop muscle! Next up comes that tablespoon of honey, which is best for providing energy both slowly and quickly.

This really has a specific advantage while you sleep due to the fact that you require energy while you sleep in order to delight in the best recovery. One reason a great deal of us get up feeling unhealthy and dazed (aside from the previously mentioned caffeine withdrawal), is that we have such low blood glucose. If you remember how rough you feel when you have not consumed anything for some time, picture how your body needs to feel after not consuming anything for 8 hours! Honey can resolve this issue by guaranteeing you have a stable supply throughout the night and a number of health authors strongly suggest it right prior to bed.

Cherries are also good since-- aside from being fantastic sources of vitamin C and outstanding anti-oxidants-- they likewise offer us with a natural source of melatonin. And if melatonin recognizes, it's most likely due to the fact that it is known as the 'sleep hormone.' This is what the brain generates to get us prepared for bed and it can, therefore, make us drop off to sleep quicker and additionally delight in a much deeper rest when we ultimately get there!

Why is kiwi in here? Well, really, it is selected for its synergistic impacts with the banana and peanut butter. Throughout these 3 components, we have adequate sources of magnesium, zinc and vitamin B6-- the very same components that comprise the popular supplement ZMA. ZMA is a supplement that is utilized by professional athletes to urge much deeper sleep and likewise to generate more testosterone. The zinc and magnesium are going to likewise likely have effective useful impacts on 'brain plasticity'-- simply put, they are going to assist your brain to rewire itself and create brand-new connections, binding whatever you learned throughout the day!

Hangover Smoothie

The above smoothie is going to additionally work extremely well as a hangover fix, or you can streamline it and simply utilize the most crucial components:

- Banana
- Peanut butter
- Honey

Actually, I would suggest that you do this and additionally substitute the milk with water. Milk is not extremely friendly after a hangover as it can curdle in the stomach and make you gag. Include a little bit of lemon and salt as well, to make this:

- Banana
- Peanut butter
- Water
- Honey
- Pinch of lemon
- Pinch of salt

The other 3 components, however, are best for making you feel far better after a huge night out. First of all, the bananas are going to supply you with a natural alkaline. This is going to assist to combat the undesirable results of the level of acidity in the stomach and supply a natural antacid. Great start. Simultaneously though, it is going to additionally assist you to renew your potassium. Boosting potassium is really essential as you are going to have lost your electrolytes from drinking. This is partially what is triggering your headaches. This is additionally why you should add a little bit of salt to ensure that you get the potassium and sodium balance back up to scratch-- it's a little like consuming an isotonic sports drink! Next up is the honey, which is unbelievable for hangovers. Yes, it is going to enhance your blood glucose and provide you some much-needed energy. However, at the same time, it is going to additionally supply you with a method to combat acetaldehyde.

Acetaldehyde is the primary harmful compound that the body produces when it breaks down alcohol-- this is exactly what is triggering most of your signs and it has to go. Do you know what eliminates acetaldehyde? Fructose! The water, on the other hand, is going to rehydrate you, while the protein in the peanut butter is going to assist you to renew your neurotransmitters and additionally do away with those munchies!

How to Make a Smoothie For Better Food Digestion

Why consume a smoothie to enhance food digestion? Naturally, this could be valuable if you have any food digestion problems that result in heartburn and so on, however, it's likewise simply an excellent idea for your basic health. All those nutrients you're obtaining via your smoothies are just going to be any usage if you can, in fact, absorb them and place them into action. And regrettably, a great deal of us have bad digestive function and struggle with this. That's especially accurate if you are somebody who experiences a great deal of tension in their life. The reason that stress stops food digestion is since tension triggers blood circulation to be directed towards the parts that are deemed crucial for survival.

These consist of the likes of the brain, muscles, and the senses-- however, not food digestion or immunity. What's more, is that we need a great deal of specific things in our diet plan so as to have the ability to absorb food correctly, and a lot of us simply aren't getting these important things. For instance, specific fruits are going to include enzymes that naturally assist you in breaking down foods. Among the best-known instances of this is pineapple, which includes bromelain (which is likewise great for your teeth!). At the same time, fermented foods, raw veggies and things such as yogurt are practical since they consist of live cultures of 'friendly germs.' They're described as friendly germs since they have beneficial roles in the body, consisting of the capability to produce a great deal of essential micronutrients and to assist us to develop digestion enzymes. If you believe you require a little bit of assistance with your food digestion, then attempt making a smoothie which contains any of the following components, all of which have extremely favorable impacts on food digestion:

- Pineapple

- Pear

- Melon

- Watermelon

- Hami Melon

- Papaya

- Orange

- Tangerine

- Mango

- Cauliflower

- Guava

- Tomato

- Spinach

- Chinese Yam

- Pumpkin

- Cabbage

- Sugarcane

- Grape

- Catnip

- Grapefruit

- Probiotics like fermented foods and yogurt.

This time, I am going to leave the accurate mix up to you! This is a fantastic option, though, for creating a green smoothie that is going to likewise be low in sugar and supply you with great deals of additional nutrients.

Chapter 7: Smoothies for Weight-loss, Bodybuilding and Functionality

Smoothies can aid with virtually every element of your health, which consists of improving functionality for gym rats and other individuals thinking about slimming down or putting on muscle. If you desire a smoothie that is going to take you beyond simply being 'healthy', these are a few of the very best possibilities for reaching your weight loss objectives.

The Cross Country Smoothie

The cross country smoothie can assist you to obtain more out of your runs and enhance your functionality in all types of aerobic workout. The exact components are:

- 1 cup of coconut water

- 1 cup of frozen blueberries

- 2 medium frozen bananas

- 2 tbs chia seeds

- 1 beat

- Pinch of salt

This mix has a lot of various advantages that are going to assist you to run quicker and further and lose more weight as a result-- a few of which you'll currently be really acquainted with. We have actually seen that beats aid to enhance vasodilation, for instance, to assist you to get more oxygen and blood around the body for weight-loss. We have actually likewise seen that coconut oil (and therefore water) can supply you with a lot of energy in the form of ketones.

The decision to utilize water instead of milk is essential to stop bloating and to keep you feeling light. Simply make certain that you provide yourself a lot of time before you go for the run-- preferably consume this around an hour prior to going out. Then there are the blueberries which are going to sustain you with vitamin C and the bananas which supply lots of excellent, functional energy. You may likewise have actually presumed that the bananas and salt remain in there to renew electrolytes as you run and to prevent cramping.

All that remains is the chia. Chia seeds are some remarkable seeds that have the capability to hold numerous times their volume of water. You can then eat them, and they are going to gradually launch all of that fluid within the stomach. What makes this so remarkable is that it permits you to have a constant supply of hydration as you run. If you have actually ever heard about the 'Tarahumara Tribe'-- a tribe of individuals who are understood to run marathons on an extremely routine basis-- then it may intrigue you to understand that chia seeds are believed to be among the secrets to their incredible capabilities!

Bodybuilding Smoothie

- 1 scoop of chocolate protein shake

- 2 cups entire milk

- 2 tablespoons peanut butter

- 1/2 a banana

- Kiwi

- Cherries

- 1 tablespoon honey

This is that identical smoothie we had for sleep, however, with the inclusion of the protein shake. Once again, you are going to likely wish to select whey protein, which is going to launch easily into the blood stream and which originates from milk, and is really natural and healthy. Consume this smoothie directly after an exercise, and you'll renew your muscles by supplying the amino acids they require to fix micro-tears brought on by training. What's more, is that the sugar in the smoothie is going to head directly to the muscles to bring back glycogen-- instead of being kept as fat.

Even better, consume this smoothie right before bed, and you'll have another anabolic window where you'll see boosted muscle development. In this case, however, you might wish to utilize a casein protein rather than whey. Casein releases protein far more gradually and this, in turn, suggests that it is going to supply a consistent supply as you are sleeping.

Fat Burning Smoothie

How can a smoothie loaded with sugar potentially assist you to slim down? Read the components, and after that, we'll get down to the mechanics of how this one functions.

The crucial components are:

- 1 green apple

- A handful of spinach

- 1 leaf kale

- 2 kiwi

- 1/2 cup of fresh apple juice

- 1 banana

- Pinch of ground cayenne pepper

- Macha tea

- Lemon juice

To start, this is a veggie smoothie that is going to supply you with much less sugar for each glass and consequently be less most likely to cause fat storage. This is one for those who are fretted about their teeth too! On the other hand, the apple that is present is going to supply you with vitamin C. Vitamin C is essential because-- as we have actually seen-- it can boost serotonin. What we didn't discuss about serotonin, however, is that it assists in reducing the appetite!

On the other hand, the macha tea, lemon juice and cayenne pepper are all thermogenic somewhat. That suggests they really raise your metabolic process to assist you to burn more calories during the day. If you can utilize this smoothie rather than having your routine breakfast, you ought to discover that it does a lot of good to assist you to burn through calories. This is particularly real if you have it within thirty minutes of getting up-- the spinach is going to provide you with a great quantity of protein and research studies reveal that consuming protein as quickly as you awaken can result in weight-loss!

Conclusion of Green Smoothie Cleanss

Now you have a complete understanding of why smoothies are so essential for your health and how you can utilize them to boost your immune strength, weight loss and more! Ensure that you do not take in more than one a day and that you utilize the ideas supplied to really make them suit your way of life. Consider what the outcomes are that you desire from your smoothie and make a couple of combinations that you can utilize to get all the various advantages you need. That may be much better food digestion, weight loss, much better sleep, or all of the above!

And obviously, you ought to change your smoothies and have various mixes to make the most of the variety in your eating plan. That stated, you ought to additionally make certain to keep returning to the identical smoothies and identical components to make sure that you get the long term advantages of having a great deal of nutrients and anti-oxidants.

You'll discover that whatever your selection, you begin to rapidly feel more healthier and energized. Your state of mind is going to enhance, you are going to lose fat, and you'll establish a healthy radiance that you simply can't obtain from supplements. Obviously, for finest outcomes, integrate this with a healthy way of life and training routine! However, you will not believe simply how transformative these impacts are. You're going to need to, in fact, give it a go

I hope that you enjoyed reading through this book and that you have found it useful. If you want to share your thoughts on this book, you can do so by leaving a review on the Amazon page. Have a great rest of the day.

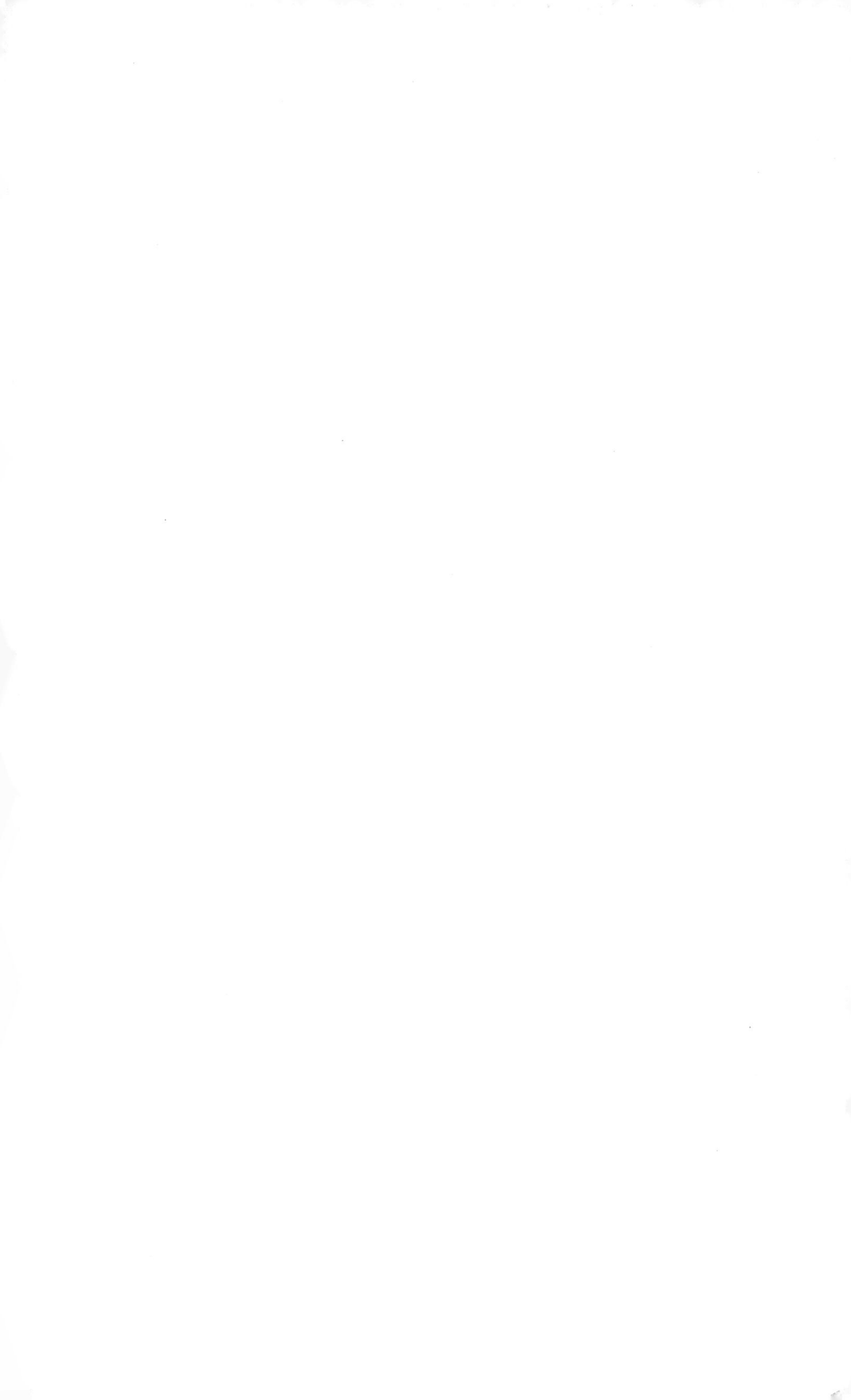

Printed in Great Britain
by Amazon